## PSYCHOLOGY AND HEALTH SERIES

Edited by Donald Marcer
Department of Psychology, University of Southampton

During the last 20 years the behavioural sciences have come to play an increasingly important part in the training of doctors, nurses and other health professionals. Not surprisingly, this shift of emphasis in education has been accompanied by a minor deluge of textbooks, all concerned with the relationship of psychology to health. Though many of these books are excellent, the range of subject matter that most of them seek to encompass necessarily means that many complex issues cannot be covered at anything other than a superficial level.

This series consists of individual texts, each dealing in some depth with a particular issue in which health professionals and psychologists have a shared interest. Though most are written by psychologists with an established academic record, they are aimed primarily at practising professionals. With this in mind, the contributing authors have all had experience in teaching students or members of the medical and other health professions and, with very few exceptions, have worked in a clinical setting. They are thus well suited to fulfil the brief that is common to all the books in this series: that is, while the theoretical basis of the issue under discussion must be spelt out, it must be done in such a way that it enables readers (be they doctors, nurses, physiotherapists, etc., or students) to practise their professions more effectively.

1. Biofeedback and Related Therapies in Clinical Practice
   *Donald Marcer*
2. Psychological Problems in Primary Health Care
   *Eric Button*
3. Psychology and Diabetes
   Psychosocial factors in management and control
   *Richard W. Shillitoe*
4. Communicating with Patients
   Improving communication, satisfaction and compliance
   *Philip Ley*
5. Understanding Stress
   A psychological perspective for health professionals
   *Valerie J. Sutherland and Cary L. Cooper*
6. Psychosexual Therapy
   A cognitive–behavioural approach
   *Susan H. Spence*
7. The Emotional and Sexual Lives of Older People
   A manual for professionals
   *H.B. Gibson*

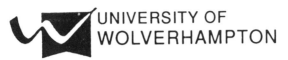

# FORTHCOMING TITLES

**Breaking Bad News?**
Giving diagnoses to patients
*Ian Robinson*

**Family Systems in Health and Illness**
*Arlene Vetere*

# The Emotional and Sexual Lives of Older People

## A MANUAL FOR PROFESSIONALS

## H.B. Gibson

*Honorary Senior Research Fellow*
*Hatfield Polytechnic*
*Hatfield, UK*

**CHAPMAN & HALL**

London · New York · Tokyo · Melbourne · Madras

**Published by Chapman & Hall, 2–6 Boundary Row, London SE1 8HN**

---

Chapman & Hall, 2–6 Boundary Row, London SE1 8HN, UK

Chapman & Hall, 29 West 35th Street, New York NY10001, USA

Chapman & Hall Japan, Thomson Publishing Japan, Hirakawacho Nemoto Building, 7F, 1-7-11 Hirakawa-cho, Chiyoda-ku, Tokyo 102, Japan

Chapman & Hall Australia, Thomas Nelson Australia, 102 Dodds Street, South Melbourne, Victoria 3205, Australia

Chapman & Hall India, R. Seshadri, 32 Second Main Road, CIT East, Madras 600 035, India

---

First edition 1992

© 1992 Chapman & Hall

Typeset in 10/12pt Times by Excel Typesetters Company, Hong Kong
Printed in Great Britain by Page Bros, Norfolk

ISBN 0 412 39360 3

The publisher makes no representation, express or implied, with regard to the accuracy of the information contained in this book and cannot accept any legal responsibility or liability for any errors or omissions that may be made.

A catalogue record for this book is available from the British Library

Library of Congress Cataloging-in-Publication data
Gibson, H.B. (Hamilton Bertie)
    The emotional and sexual lives of older people: a manual for professionals / H.B. Gibson. – 1st ed.
        p.      cm. – (Psychology and health series; 7)
    Includes bibliographical references and index.
    ISBN 0–412–39360–3
        1. Gerontology. 2. Geriatrics. 3. Aged–Sexual behavior.
    4. Love in old age. I. Title. II. Series: Psychology and health series; v. 7.
    HQ1061.G45   1991
    306.7′084′6–dc20                                   91–24470
                                                          CIP

# Contents

# Acknowledgements

I am happy to acknowledge the help of a number of eminent specialists in gerontology and related disciplines, both through their published work and their personal communications. Two tables (1.3 and 6.3) are reprinted from pp. 172 and 313 of *Love, Sex and Aging: A Consumers Union Report* by Edward M. Brecher and the Editors of Consumer Report Books by permission of Little, Brown and Company. The work of Robert N. Butler and Myrna I. Lewis has provided a constant inspiration and I have frequently referred to their publications; similarly, I owe much to Alex Comfort who originally gave me the idea for the book. I have quoted freely from Lesley H. Croft's *Sexuality in Later Life*, and she and her publishers, Butterworth Heinemann, have kindly given permission for the reprinting of the material that appears in Appendix B of her book. Like all writers in this field, I owe much to the original studies of A.C. Kinsey and his colleagues; I have frequently referred to their pioneer work and to that of William H. Masters and Virginia E. Johnson whose names appear frequently in this book. Among the important research studies which I have drawn upon is the Duke University Study of Human Aging and I am indebted to Eric Pfeiffer for his permission to quote from it. *The Starr–Weiner Report*, which was originally published by McGraw-Hill, has also been a fertile source of research material and Bernard D. Starr has kindly allowed me to reproduce two of the tables. Another important table, which appeared in *The Aging Experience*, is that of Russell A. Ward, and he and his publishers, J.B. Lippincott Co., have given their permission for its reproduction.

Various institutions and associations have contributed to this book by their co-operation, particularly: the Centre for Policy on Ageing, whose librarian, Gillian Crosby, has been especially helpful; Age Concern with their invaluable pamphlets; and The University of the Third Age in Cambridge who have given permission for the reproduction of a table from their publication *The Image of the Elderly on TV*. In my survey of the training of nurses, clinical psychologists, medical students and social workers, I am indebted to a large number of specialists in these fields who have contributed in presenting a coherent picture. Although all those who have helped me so generously are too numerous to list I must mention, in addition to the above, some specialists whose names will be familiar to most of those working in the field of gerontology/geriatric medicine whose assistance has been particularly helpful: John Anderson, Jennie Bright, Martin Cole, Peter Coleman, Nicholas Coni, Gian Degun, Malcolm Johnson, Christine Kalus, John Kellett, Michael Lye, Niel McKenzie, Alistair Main, Pauline Newson, Alison Norman, Jane Palmer, Robert Stout, Cameron Swift and Archie Young. A number of these have read portions of the manuscript in draft and made useful comments and suggestions.

In addition to acknowledging the help given to me by all these people from their various professional backgrounds, I would like to thank Rosemary Morris, the Senior Editor in Health Sciences of my publishers, whose assistance and encouragement have contributed to the writing of the book. I must also acknowledge the patient help given by my daughter Jennifer Gibson in the technical production of the indexes.

Finally, my greatest debt is to Carol Graham with whom I have discussed every aspect of the book as it has been written. Not only has she read and corrected the whole manuscript, and contributed much to its stylistic presentation, but it is to her that I owe so many of the ideas that are developed in this book.

H.B. Gibson

# Introduction

Professional people such as doctors, clinical psychologists, counsellors, social workers, nurses and priests are becoming increasingly concerned with the emotional needs of people over the age of retirement. Many of us are now aware that in our original professional training, insufficient attention was paid to matters that are very much to the fore in current practice. GPs and others are now being asked by older patients about emotional and sexual matters that used not to be discussed so frankly or so frequently. Various bodies such as Age Concern are encouraging the 'new old' to expect to lead fuller lives, and to seek the help and advice of professional workers in health care about matters that were frequently overlooked in former times.

This book is written with the object of helping people in the health-care professions to become fully aware of the great wealth of information that is now available about the processes of ageing from psychological, medical, sociological, and demographic sources. The great change in the population structure, with many more people living into the later decades of life, is a tendency that is world wide, but is most pronounced in the Western world. There, improvements in public health have been most advanced in the present century, and there has been an historically early adoption of a policy of family limitation that has skewed the age distribution towards the upper end.

The present cohorts of people who were born in the first third of this century – those who are over 60 years of age now in the 1990s – experienced in their younger years the educative and formative influences of a society that was very different from that which developed after World War II. Technological change has been matched by quite profound changes in social attitudes. The older people of today were brought up by parents and parental figures who were themselves strongly influenced by an ethos that is often characterized as 'Victorian'. That Victorian values had certain merits is not debated here; we are simply concerned with the fact that in that era 'the old' were regarded very differently from how they are beginning to be regarded in modern times, and from the image they are now striving to create for themselves.

Public attitudes towards a number of important aspects of human behaviour, including the expression of sexuality, have changed very radically, and in considering the total emotional adjustment of older people today, this book discusses love and sexuality in later life, in its broadest sense. This is an era of transition for people who are now in the 'Third Age', and professional people are necessarily concerned with a wide range of problems that have arisen.

It is instructive to consider the factors that have brought the question of love and sex in later life into prominence in recent years. In the post-war era the studies of Kinsey produced quite a revolution in thinking about the sex lives of young and middle-aged adults, and the re-adjustment of social values led to the later inquiries of a more detailed nature, notably the clinical studies of Masters and Johnson. Such studies tended to operate on the erroneous assumption that it was hardly worth while inquiring about, or being concerned with, men and women over the age of 60. In the past, people in this age-group seldom consulted their doctors or other health-care professionals about sexual problems, and so it was assumed that normal older people were totally uninterested in sex.

The decade of the 1970s saw a proliferation of different sorts of books dealing with sex, and much of the older folk-lore that served rather repressive attitudes was disconfirmed by more rational inquiries. Most of these books hardly touched on the love and sex-lives of senior citizens. Towards the end of that decade, however, increasing factual knowledge about the sex-lives of older people began to be recognized in scientific circles. There was the Starr-Weiner Report published in 1981, and Edward Brecher's study for the American Consumers' Association, reporting on the sex lives of 4,246 men and women aged between 50 and 93, was published in 1984. The social and medical implications of these findings are coming to be recognized, and a good deal of re-thinking is going on in scientific circles. We now recognize that many normal men and women in their 60s, 70s and older do indeed have significant sex lives both emotionally and physically, although expressed rather differently than in their younger years. Some of these people are in greater need of the help and advice of professionals than are younger adults.

The facts that have emerged may surprise many of us. When

people reach an age that society designates as 'old', many are themselves surprised to find that they do not feel any different, except for an inevitable waning of their physical robustness. Individuals who are conscious that they still have the same emotional and physical reactions sexually, including those in relation to their own long-standing marital partners, may privately regard themselves as being rather 'odd', and may fail to realize that they are entirely normal. At first they may feel very diffident about admitting the reality of their emotional and sexual feelings to professional care-givers, but when the latter can reassure them concerning the true facts about others in their age-group, and older, then they begin to realize that ageing as such need not make a very great difference to their needs and feelings in this respect. If this realization is achieved, it produces a great increase in self-confidence, and heartens people to fulfil their true potential in the later years. As yet we lack sufficient hard data about the relationship of continued health and longevity to emotional and sexual satisfaction, but there are some encouraging pointers.

This book discusses how professional workers can assist people to continue to get the best out of life in the later years, with love and sex playing the part that is normal in adulthood, and recognizing the extent of individual differences. As was shown in the Kinsey Reports, it is difficult to set a norm for sexual behaviour and experience, and increasingly we are becoming aware of the impossibility of defining what is to be expected at any particular age. However, a great deal of reliable information concerning the physiological changes that take place with ageing and the psychological and social factors that interact with such age-related changes is now available. The first two chapters of this book describe in some detail what is known of the normal sexual responses of men and women, and how the natural processes of ageing affect these responses. Common difficulties that may arise with ageing are discussed, and it is pointed out how professional people may provide relevant advice and counselling.

The third chapter deals with the implications of society's image of older people and the stereotypes that are a relic of the past. In particular, the question of the 'survival curve' is discussed: this is a model of ageing based upon findings that, contrary to widespread assumptions, most people's health and well-being do not steadily and progressively decline in the later years until the point of death, but that, given adequate social and medical support, vigour and independence can be maintained for practically the whole of the life-span.

Public stereotypes of ageing are changing, but they still affect how people regard themselves as they grow older, and create problems in the achievement of a satisfactory emotional adjustment. Professional people are not immune from the influence of a powerful mythology about the elderly that has been the subject of a sustained attack by pioneers such as Edward Brecher, Robert Butler, Alex Comfort, Myrna Lewis, Alison Norman, and Bernard Starr in recent years, and whose work is cited extensively in this book. A wide range of facts, the product of recent research in the different disciplines that contribute to gerontology, has to be considered in arriving at a realistic appreciation of the needs of older people, and how social policies should contribute to their well-being. That professional workers in the different health-care disciplines need to examine carefully their role in this matter, and the training they give to students, is discussed in Chapter 4. Here we have the problem that not only must students be required to learn a great deal of factual information about their own profession, and kindred professions, but their attitudes to the elderly need to be considered, and, in some cases, modified through extensive discussion and exposure to other means of education.

The various kinds of problems that may arise in families are discussed in Chapter 5. The upheavals occasioned by changing social circumstances and modifications in social attitudes are considered. Younger people sometimes exhibit a double standard of morality: a permissive set of attitudes to those of their own generation, and a more restrictive one to those in their parents' generation. Occasionally there are mercenary motives for seeking to restrict the freedom of the older members of their family, and a wish to exploit their labour, coupled with a desire to conserve very carefully all money that forms an inheritance. Situations that produce actual violence against older relatives are also described, and some remedies are proposed.

Emotional stresses in later life that have a broadly sexual basis are considered in Chapter 6. Retirement from work may precipitate problems in the readjustment of the sex-roles, and the various changes that accompany ageing may produce sexual difficulties in marriages that have previously been harmonious.

Older people living in different types of retirement homes present special problems in the relations between the sexes that call for understanding and skilful management on the part of professional people. The question of the changing expression of sexuality with ageing is further discussed in Chapter 7, where it is suggested that sex education for later life is, for many people, as important as education in this matter for children. Many people enter the 'Third Age' rather ignorant of what to expect regarding their own sexuality and that of their partner, and burdened with a great deal of misinformation, the legacy of past myths that even had the sanction of some medical opinion. Professional workers can help to dispel these myths, and assist people to achieve a more realistic understanding of how they can best adjust to changes in themselves and their partners.

The question of the general health of older people is considered in Chapter 8, and the 'survival curve' mentioned in Chapter 3 is further discussed in relation to the question of longevity. Research has suggested that in maintaining vigour and independence throughout the span of life, subjectively perceived health is of primary importance. The medical assessment of health does not always predict continued fitness and longevity as effectively as the 'quality of life', a variable that is difficult to define. The nature of some common disabilities that are associated with ageing are discussed, and related to the remedial measures that professional workers can implement.

In the final chapter we attempt to look ahead to the twenty-first century and examine some probable and possible developments in the status of older people in society. This leads to some speculation in the fields of social security, medicine, marriage and sexuality. It is evident that the very oldest section of the population will increase numerically more than other age cohorts in the next two decades, and this has some important implications for social policy. The great numerical disparity between men and women in the later decades of life is not likely to diminish significantly in the foreseeable future, and this raises some important problems that need to be examined, particularly with regard to the institution of marriage. It is argued that such speculation is justified by the need continually to examine our current practices, and to study how to modify them in the face of changing circumstances.

# 1

# The physiology of age-related changes in sexual capacity and experience: a plan for therapy. I Men

In both sexes, the normal process of ageing brings about certain changes in sexual capacity and the emotional and sensory experience of sexuality. This is to be expected, for many of the body's functions change as we age. In our sixties we no longer expect to run as fast as we did in our twenties even if we are perfectly healthy, and in more subtle ways the body changes in its resistance to stress and disease. The general decline in our physical powers has led to a false belief that sexuality, both in terms of performance, needs and interest, should normally fade out somewhere in the late fifties, and that if it persists it may take pathological forms. Thus Havelock Ellis (1933) popularized the idea that there was something abnormal and potentially dangerous in older people remaining sexually active. He wrote:

> There is a frequent well marked tendency in women at the menopause to an eruption of sexual desire, the last flaring up of a dying fire, which may easily take on a morbid form.
>
> Similarly in men, when the approach of age begins to be felt, the sexual impulse may become suddenly urgent. In this instinctive reaction it may tend to roam, normally or abnormally, beyond legitimate bounds. . . . This late exacerbation of sexuality becomes still more dangerous if it takes the form of an attraction to girls who are no more than children, and to acts of indecent familiarity with children. . . . the average age of the victim regularly decreases as the average age of the perpetrator increases (Ellis, 1933, pp. 181–182).

Subsequent research has shown that Havelock Ellis' statement on this matter has no foundation in fact. He goes on to perpetuate the mischievous myth that sexual interest in later life presages senile dementia, stating that:

> with physical irritation, such as may arise from an enlarged prostate, and with psychic loss of control from incipient mental decay, there is a risk that the barriers may be removed, and the man become a danger to himself and to others. It is in this way sometimes that senile dementia begins to declare itself before intellectual failure is obvious (Ellis, 1933, p. 182).

There is no evidence that enlargement of the prostate has such an effect. In fact, sexuality is less affected by ageing than many other functions of the body, particularly for the female sex, although the procreative ability of the latter ceases with the menopause around the age of 50, with considerable inter-individual differences. Emotionally, we probably change less with age than physically, but our emotional life is very much influenced by many factors, including our upbringing and the culture and environment in which we live. What is very important for the whole area of the physical and emotional expression of love and sexuality at all ages is the self-image of the individual, and considerable inportance will be given to this topic throughout the present book.

This manual is directed to health-care professionals of all kinds, and although some professionals such as social workers are not directly concerned with the medical details of conditions affecting their clients' health and general functioning, it is essential that they should be fully aware of the physiological facts, just as physicians should be fully aware of the social and psychological factors that are involved in all aspects of ageing.

Granted that people's sexual activity is very much determined by their general outlook and their emotional lives, we may examine the extent to which sexual expression, needs and interests are influenced by the sheer physical changes that take place with age. Here we shall discriminate between changes that are normal (i.e. usual in the ageing but healthy body) and those that are the result of degenerative disease processes that may attack us with increasing frequency as we age. Because research has shown that the two sexes age very differently as regards sexual capacity and expression, they will be discussed separately in these first two chapters.

## THE NORMAL SEXUAL EXPERIENCE AND BEHAVIOUR OF OLDER MEN

The well-known studies of Kinsey *et al.* (1948) indicated a steady decline in the frequency of sexual activity throughout the life span of men, leading to 'more or less permanent erectile impotence' in 27% of men by the age of 70 years. According to later researchers, this figure is a gross over-estimate. The Kinsey studies suffered from a number of features that make their conclusions about older people unreliable. First, the studies were cross-sectional, that is, separate age-groups were studied over a wide age range. Thus the differences between these age-groups may partly have been due to the altered circumstances under which older and younger generations had grown up. It is therefore likely that men in the older age-groups were rather more reticent about their sex-lives, whatever their actual habits were, as befitted the conventions under which they had been reared. Kinsey's 80-year-olds were born around 1880. However, the results were interpreted as though they had come from a longitudinal survey, that is, the same people being studied over a continuous period of their development. George and Weiler (1981) studied their samples of middle-aged and older people for six years, and came to the conclusion that the effects due to generational differences were greater than those due to ageing.

A further aspect of the Kinsey studies of both men and women should be noted; there were very few older people represented. Starr (1985) notes that:

> one of the most powerful statements that Kinsey made about the status of sex and aging is the number of pages he devoted to the subject: four pages on older women and three pages on older men, out of 1,646 pages in his two volumes (Starr, 1985, p. 100).

Kinsey's total number of subjects was 12,000, but the number of people over 60 years was only 186, a totally inadequate sample. Croft (1982) also points out that in the influential studies of Masters and Johnson (1966) the number of older people was rather small and therefore somewhat unreliable in terms of what we may conclude about the effect of ageing on sexuality. Finally, it should be noted that in the Kinsey study of men, sexual behaviour was defined as activity that culminates in orgasm.

3

Normally when we speak of orgasm in men we mean a seminal emission accompanied by a sudden neurological climax. However, in older men this neurological event, the climax, may not be accompanied by any seminal emission on all, or any, occasions, hence there is some ambiguity in the literature about the meaning of the term 'orgasm'. Comfort (1990) obviously implies a seminal emission and ejaculation when he writes, 'Ageing induces some changes in human sexual performance. These are chiefly in the male, for whom orgasm becomes less frequent. It occurs in every second act of intercourse, or in one act in three, rather than every time' (p. 60). However, Comfort is writing here for the lay public; other authorities go into some detail regarding the culmination of the sex act. Bancroft (1983) specifies three separate events: emission, ejaculation, and orgasm. He observes that 'The relationship between these three components remains obscure, except that they usually occur together' (p. 60).

In this connection we should note that Dunn and Trost (1989) studied men who have a 'non-ejaculatory orgasm' and cultivate the ability to have repeated orgasms without ejaculation, an ability that increases with age. Robbins and Jensen (1978) also write of repeated orgasms without ejaculation, except for the final orgasm that produces ejaculation. It seems entirely arbitrary to adopt the Kinsey definition of 'sexual activity' and to exclude from the category all acts of lovemaking, even peno-vaginal intercourse, that do not culminate in seminal ejaculation. In the present book, orgasm in the male will be considered more on a par with such an event in the female, a neurophysiological climax that is popularly known as 'coming', whether or not any semen is emitted from the male. Kinsey compared the neurological aspect of the orgasm to an epileptic fit, and there is indeed some later EEG evidence that makes such a comparison valid (Heath, 1972). According to Fisher et al. (1983) the neurophysiological event of orgasm involves the release of circuits in the lateral hypothalamus from higher limbic areas and cortical regions.

Some years before Havelock Ellis published his book, more reliable factual material about the sex-lives of older people was already available. In a 1930 study by Pearl (cited by Comfort, 1979) it was found that 4% of males in their seventies were having sexual intercourse about three times a week, and 9% were having it at least once a week. Turning to rather later studies

**Table 1.1** Reasons for the cessation of sexual relations

| Reason | Males | | Females | |
|---|---|---|---|---|
| | No. | % | No. | % |
| Death of spouse | 0 | — | 35 | 36 |
| Separation or divorce | 0 | — | 12 | 12 |
| Illness of spouse | 5 | 14 | 19 | 20 |
| Loss of interest by spouse | 3 | 9 | 4 | 4 |
| Spouse unable to perform sexually | 2 | 6 | 17 | 18 |
| Illness of self | 6 | 17 | 2 | 2 |
| Loss of interest by self | 5 | 14 | 4 | 4 |
| Self unable to perform sexually | 14 | 40 | 4 | 4 |
| Total | 35 | | 97 | |

Pfeiffer, E, Verwoerdt, A. and Davis, G. C. (1972) Sexual behavior in middle life. *Am. J. Psychiat.*, 128, 1264–1266. Reprinted by permission.

of elderly people, we get a very different picture from that portrayed by Havelock Ellis. Finkle *et al.* (1959) questioned 101 healthy men between the ages of 56 and 86 and found that 65% under the age of 69 years, and 34% of those over the age of 70 years were still sexually active, with two out of five over 80 averaging at least ten acts of sexual intercourse a year. In the research of Bretschneider and McCoy (1981), who studied the sexual interest and behaviour of healthy people between the ages of 80 and 102 years, 62% of male residents in retirement homes in California had recently had sexual intercourse, and 87% had had recent physical sexual intimacy of some kind. The figures for the elderly women in their study were respectively 30% and 68%, but in the community studied there were six women to every man!

There is some evidence that when sexual activity ceases, even in middle-age, it is more likely to be due to incapacity on the part of the male rather than the female partner. This is exemplified in a study by Pfeiffer *et al.* (1972), the results of which are shown in Table 1.1.

It will be seen that the most common reason for women ceasing to have sexual relations (36% of the sample) was that their spouse had died, and that relatively few women were prevented by their own illness, loss of interest or incapacity. In contrast, the most frequent reason for men ceasing to be sexually active (40% of the sample) was their own inability to perform. However, too much attention must not be paid to the high rate of disability shown in this study because it was a *medical* study, and many of the subjects were people seeking medical care because of various infirmities.

In more recent years there have been a number of large surveys of the sexual lives of older people, and they have indicated that, whatever may have been true in the past, older people are now much more sexually active that was previously believed. How do we account for the discrepancy between the rather conservative estimates of sexual activity among older people that used to be found, and the more liberal estimates coming from modern research? According to Starr (1985):

> the discrepancy between earlier findings of low levels of sexual activity and interest among the elderly and recent findings to the contrary is that earlier studies were guided by the prevailing self-fulfilling prophesy – little sex was expected and consequently little was found. Researchers were even discouraged from pursuing the topic in the belief that older people would be resistant or unresponsive to sexual queries . . . or that their adult children would stop them from participating in such research (Starr, 1985, p. 99).

Starr goes on to point out that nowadays older people are living much more independent lives, and that their adult children have little control over what they do. He also mentions the research artefact referred to above in the Kinsey studies, and calls attention to the unrepresentative nature of the sample studied by Pfeiffer *et al.* (1972).

Starr and Weiner (1981) used a 50-item questionnaire that required subjects to write answers to open-ended questions about a broad range of topics referring to their sexual lives. This was given to a population of 800 people over the age of 60 years, 282 males and 518 females. The results were analysed and expressed as 50 tables and additional sub-tables, showing the responses of males and females separately. In some cases the tables were broken down into age groups, 60–69 years, 70–79 years, and 80–91 years, thus showing how people differed over a span of 31 years, differences being due to both physiological and attitudinal factors. A typical table from the appendix of this Report is shown in Table 1.2.

**Table 1.2** How often do you have sexual relations?

| CATEGORY | TOTALS | | MALES | | FEMALES | |
|---|---|---|---|---|---|---|
| | All Subjects | Adjusted | All Subjects | Adjusted | All Subjects | Adjusted |
| When in the Mood | 43 | | 17 | | 26 | |
| | (5.4%) | (6.1%) | (6.0%) | (6.5%) | (5.0%) | (5.9%) |
| Three Times a | 85 | | 39 | | 46 | |
| Week or More | (10.6) | (12.1) | (13.8) | (14.9) | (8.9) | (10.4) |
| Twice a Week | 93 | | 43 | | 50 | |
| | (11.6) | (13.2) | (15.2) | (16.5) | (9.6) | (11.3) |
| Once a Week | 129 | | 61 | | 68 | |
| | (16.1) | (18.3) | (21.6) | (23.4) | (13.1) | (15.4) |
| Three Times a | 7 | | 3 | | 4 | |
| Month | (0.9) | (1.0) | (1.1) | (1.1) | (0.8) | (0.9) |
| Twice a Month | 57 | | 23 | | 34 | |
| | (7.1) | (8.1) | (8.2) | (8.8) | (6.6) | (7.7) |
| Once a Month | 69 | | 29 | | 40 | |
| | (8.6) | (9.8) | (10.3) | (11.1) | (7.8) | (9.0) |
| Less than Once a | 70 | | 27 | | 43 | |
| Month | (8.8) | (10.0) | (9.6) | (10.3) | (8.3) | (9.7) |
| Not Active | 150 | | 19 | | 131 | |
| | (18.8) | (21.3) | (6.7) | (7.3) | (25.2) | (29.6) |
| No Response | 97 | | 21 | | 76 | |
| | (12.1) | | (7.5) | | (14.7) | |
| Total Responses | 800 | | 282 | | 518 | |

It will be appreciated that not every individual in the 800 sample responded to every question, and this is allowed for in the table shown by presenting 'adjusted' percentages as shown in parentheses. It may be seen from the table that of those responding, only 7.3% of males and 29.6% of females are 'not active', and these figures must be considered in the light of the fact that as we go up the age gradient, an increasing number of women are necessarily without male partners because of the differential death-rate, a matter that will be fully discussed in Chapter 6. In the sub-table dealing with these data in terms of the three age groups (not reproduced here) it may be seen that even in the 80–91-year-old group only three of the 20 males are 'not active'. As the age span is quite great, averages are somewhat misleading if we amalgamate all the groups, as shown in Table 1.2, but the authors work out the averages as follows: average frequency of sexual relations per week = 1.40 (total population); males = 1.44; females = 1.39.

Obviously these figures geve a somewhat exaggerated picture of the frequency of sexual intercourse among people over the age of 60 years, as 12.1% of the sample did not answer this question, and this minority probably includes a great number of those who are sick, disabled, alone and otherwise debarred from sexual relations, as well as those who just did not feel like answering this question. The Starr-Weiner Report on the sex-lives of 800 people is therefore mainly concerned with giving us a picture of how *healthy* people behave despite the growing physiological weaknesses that come with age, and we must not be confused by the findings of the various medical studies that have been concerned with patient populations and consequently show much lower rates of sexual activity.

Another large study that can be compared with that of Starr and Weiner was carried out by Brecher (1984) on behalf of the American Consumers' Union. It was carried out in 1978/79, and concerned the emotional and sexual lives of 4,246 people (2,402 men and 1,844 women) in the age range 50–93 years, and asked an enormous range of questions dealing not only with what people did, but what their attitudes were to a great number of topics relevant to love and sex in later life. Because of the great age range covered (43 years) the findings have to be expressed separately at different age levels, and for the purpose of this chapter it will suffice to say little more than that the study amply confirmed all that had been found in the Starr-Weiner Report. Because of the very great number of the respondents to the Brecher study, respondents who were mainly in good health, it is very important for the purpose of the present book, and in relation to the present chapter it is worth quoting the following:

Our 4,246 respondents constitute the largest geriatric sample ever assembled for a sexuality study – not only for the total period after the age 50 but also for each decade from the fifties through the eighties. Our sample is the first one large enough to permit charting sexual changes between the fifties and the sixties, and between the sixties and subsequent years – for women and for men separately.

**Table 1.3** The decline of sexual activity with age

|                 | In their 50s | In their 60s | Aged 70 and over |
| --------------- | ------------ | ------------ | ---------------- |
| All women       | (N = 801)    | (N = 719)    | (N = 324)        |
| Sexually active | 93%          | 81%          | 65%              |
| All men         | (N = 823)    | (N = 981)    | (N = 598)        |
| Sexually active | 98%          | 91%          | 79%              |

Reprinted from *Love, Sex and Aging: A Consumers Union Report* by Edward M. Brecher and the Editors of Consumer Reports Books, p. 313. Copyright © 1984 by Consumers Union of the United States, Inc. By permission of Little, Brown and Company.

Our two central findings can be stated with confidence:
Male sexual function undergoes a gradual, steady decline from the fifties on.
Female sexual function also undergoes a decline from the fifties on. (Brecher, 1984 pp. 312–313).

The decline of sexual activity with age in Brecher's sample is shown in Table 1.3.

It will be seen from Table 1.3 that although there is a decline in sexual activity with age, it is quite a gradual decline. The apparent greater decline in females is misleading, for, as will be shown later in this book, the decline in capacity is *less* for females, but the figures reflect the growing numerical imbalance between the sexes in the population in the later decades of life.

**The normal sexual response of the male**

Before detailing the age-related physiological changes that normally take place in the male, it will be helpful to set out very briefly a model of the responses of the younger adult male to sexual stimuli and how they culminate in intercourse, ejaculation, orgasm and final resolution. For the sake of convenience we will take the well-known model of Masters and Johnson (1966), although it was formulated 25 years ago and has been subjected to criticim and modification by later researchers such as Kaplan (1974) and Cooper (1988).

Masters and Johnson (1966) propose a four-phase sexual cycle *excitement*, *plateau*, *orgasmic* and *resolution*. They used this model also for the female sexual cycle which will be considered in Chapter 2, with some critical comments.

(i) The excitement phase: for the young man, sexual stimuli cause a pressure of blood to build up in the two cavernous cylinders of the penis, the corpora cavernosa, that lie parallel to each other, and in a third cylinder of erectile tissue, the corpus spongiosum, which contains the urethra, the head of the penis (the glans) being formed from the distal end. The suffusion of the whole organ with blood, and hence erection occurring, is caused partly by constriction of the valves controlling venous outflow, and partly by dilation of the arterioles supplying the erectile tissue. This mechanism is triggered by neural control from higher cortical centres, and also by a reflex action controlled by centres in the sacral part of the spinal cord, the whole being dependent on an appropriate balance between the sympathetic and para-sympathetic systems.

(ii) The plateau phase: in this the penis remains erect, whether or not it receives tactile stimulation, as in intercourse. In some men, this period may be prolonged for a considerable period, even though there are the strong tactile stimuli of intercourse which eventually produce orgasm.

(iii) The orgasmic phase: in Masters and Johnson's formulation, this phase is concerned with the rhythmic contractions of various structures which expel the seminal fluid. First, fluid is emitted from the seminal vesicles and other structures containing it, and builds up in the prostatic part of the urethra, and the man becomes aware that ejaculation is imminent – this is the so-called 'point of ejaculatory inevitability' which persists for 1–4 seconds. This is stage one. In stage two, in Masters and Johnson's words 'The seminal fluid is expelled the full length of the penile urethra under severe pressure created by the involuntary but co-ordinated contractions of these muscle groupings' (p. 185). They make the point that 'many men learn to restrain or delay their ejaculatory reaction until their partner is satiated'.

(iv) The resolution phase: this is presented as taking place in two stages; the first occurs very rapidly and reduces the penis to about twice the size of the normal, flaccid organ. The second occurs slowly as the penis shrinks to the normal state. A refractory period then takes place in which stimuli which previously had been excitatory produce no physiological response. The refractory period can be quite brief in some young men.

## Normal physiological changes with ageing

We can now discuss the main changes that normally take place with ageing. This is very necessary, as if men do not understand what normally takes place (a process that alters but does not abolish their sexual powers), then they fear that they are becoming 'impotent' when they notice changes taking place. Such a fear may well affect their emotional state so they suffer from a condition of psychogenic impotency that is not the result of physiological incapacity. It is therefore incumbent upon professional health-care workers who are consulted about health and happiness to have an accurate knowledge of the nature of such changes, and to forewarn men who may otherwise suffer as a result of their misunderstanding. Masters and Johnson (1970) write very feelingly of men who become needlessly obsessed with the fear of impotency:

> Tragically, yet understandably, tens of thousands of men have moved from effective sexual functioning to varying degrees of secondary impotence because they did not understand the natural variants that physiological aging imposes on previously established patterns of sexual functioning.
>
> From a psychosexual point of view, the male over 50 has to contend with one of the great fallacies of our culture. Every man in this age group is arbitrarily defined by both public and professional alike as sexually impaired. When the aging male is faced by unexplained but natural involutional sexual changes, and deflated by widespread psychosocial acceptance of the fallacy of sexual incompetence as a natural component of the aging process, is it any wonder that he carries a constantly increasing fear of sexual performance? (Masters and Johnson, 1970, p. 316).

In their discussion of the natural ageing process, Masters and Johnson use the terms 'older man' to refer to those from 50–70 years of age, and 'younger man' to describe the 20–40-year-old

11

group. They describe the age-related changes in terms of the four phases that have already been briefly outlined.

(i) Excitement phase. While the younger man often develops an erection in a matter of seconds when he responds to excitatory stimuli, it may take the older man several minutes to respond. The penis will not be as elevated or as firm as in the younger years.

(ii) Plateau phase. This phase lasts longer for the older man, and he can deliberately prolong it more easily without being troubled by the ejaculatory demand that may make the phase all too brief for some younger men who sometimes fail to satisfy their partners.

(iii) Orgasmic phase. In the young man the pattern of ejaculatory response is more or less standard and the same on all occasions. For the older man there is far more variability between occasions (and indeed, between individuals, as later researchers have found). The period of 'ejaculatory inevitability' is less noticeable in the older man, and the process of climax may be one-stage rather than two-stage as in the younger man. Alternatively, this final stage may last for as long as seven seconds, the prostate going into a prolonged spasm. There may be a considerable reduction in the amount of semen ejaculated (about 1–3 ml as compared with 3–5 ml), and it spurts out with considerably less force.

(iv) Resolution phase. This takes place far more rapidly in the older man, and there is a lessened tendency for it take place in two stages. The refractory period is longer, and so while the younger man can engage in several acts of intercourse in a night, this is seldom possible for the older man.

## ABNORMAL DISABILITIES IN THE SEXUAL FUNCTION OF AGEING MEN

It used to be generally asserted that about 90% of cases of sexual dysfunction in men were due to psychological factors, and therapists were disappointed to find how often psycho-sexual counselling was quite ineffective in restoring function, particularly with older men. Later research has shown that between 30% and 70% of erectile failures are due to organic causes (Michal, 1982; Melman et al., 1984). Fortunately, many conditions of organically

**Table 1.4** Drugs that are least likely to cause sexual dysfunction in the male

---

*ACE inhibitors*
Capotopril
Lisonopril
Enalapril maleate

*Beta blocker*
Atenolol

*Calcium channel blockers*
Nifedipine
Dilatiagem

*Anti-ulcer measures*
Ranitidine

*Antidepressants*
Fluoxetine
Trazodone*
Desipramine

*Anti-anxiety agents*
Lorazepam
Alprazolam
Buspirone

---

* Trazodone may cause priapism.
Source: Barber *et al.* (1989a) Sexual problems in the elderly, I: The use and abuse of medications. *Geriatrics,* 44, 61–71.

induced impotence are reversible. Some of the more common forms of disability will be described.

## 1 Drug-related disabilities

One of the commonest causes of lowered potency of men in their later years is the side effects of medically prescribed drugs. According to Whitehead (in Barber *et al.*, 1989a) 'There are some 200 different medicines that are used for very bonafide reasons but that affect sexual function' (p. 62). He goes on to mention the drugs that are *least likely* to cause sexual dysfunction and these are shown in Table 1.4.

At the symposium at which Dr Whitehead spoke, Dr Long

suggested that the anti-ulcer medication ranitidine had not yet been in use long enough for there to be a firm opinion about it, as all the H blockers produce the same type of basic pharmacological process. He agreed with Dr Whitehead about most of the drugs, but mentioned that the reports of the side-effects of these drugs in the literature varied greatly. The antihypertensives, with the exception of the three mentioned by Dr Whitehead, appeared to be the worst in their side-effects causing sexual dysfunction, and the antipsychotics were the next most serious. Dr Long mentioned that fluphenazine, perphenazine, and trifluoperazine were the safest antipsychotics in relation to sexual function. The antipsychotic drug thioridizine is the one that the primary physician is most likely to prescribe for an elderly person suffering from agitation, anxiety or depression, but this drug, according to Dr Long, was responsible for 49% of patients suffering from impaired ejaculation, and 44% from impotence in one series of trials.

Chlorpromazine appears to be relatively safe when given in doses under 400 mg/d; it is only when the dose gets up to 600 mg/d that there is reduced libido, and when the dosage is as high as 1000–1500 mg/d there is the full deleterious side-effect sexually as with any other phenothiazine. Dr Long endorsed Dr Whitehead's opinion that the anti-anxiety drug buspirone was among the best for avoiding sexual side-effects. Among the antidepressants he mentioned that amoxapine was reported to reduce libido and cause impotence in men in as many as 40% of patients, and it could also inhibit orgasm in women. With regard to trazadone, which Dr Whitehead had mentioned as a good antidepressant in general but somewhat rarely causing priapism, Dr Long said that such priapism might occur in 1–2% of users, and that it might cause retrograde ejaculation, that is, when the semen is forced back into the bladder.

Myrna Lewis, a social worker, colleague and co-author of Dr Butler (Butler and Lewis, 1988), who was present at the symposium, raised the question of whether lithium might actually increase libido. Dr Long explained the general position regarding antidepressant drugs. A low dose might improve sexuality because it relieved depression, but a high dose would lower sexuality because of its toxic effects, thus there were reports in the literature of lithium both raising and lowering libido.

It was also mentioned at the symposium that alpha blockers

such as prazosin and clonidine can cause sexual dysfunction, and that the diuretics often impair erections. The problem for the physician is to devise a strategy in prescribing for elderly people to cope with those suffering from hypertension, diabetes, heart disease etc. by appropriate medication, but to preserve their sexual function as far as possible. Patients should also be advised that over-use of alcohol may lead to sexual dysfunction. Older people often drink to produce relaxation and euphoria and expect it to improve their lovemaking, but, particularly for men, alcohol can act like other drugs in inhibiting sexual performance, both temporarily and on a long-term basis (Mikhailidis et al., 1983). In the words of the Porter in Shakespeare's Macbeth 'Lechery, sir, it provokes, and unprovokes; it provokes the desire, but it takes away the performance.' Butler and Lewis (1988) point out that tolerance for alcohol may decrease with age and so smaller and smaller amounts may begin to produce negative effects with regard to sexual performance. They suggest that 'older persons' should limit themselves to a maximum of 1½ ounces of hard liquor, two six-ounce glasses of wine, or three eight-ounce glasses of beer in any twenty-four hour period. Such advice must be interpreted very liberally, as individual tolerance for alcohol varies enormously, and has sometimes been built up over most of a lifetime, in contrast to the tolerance for some medically prescribed drugs which may be encountered for the first time in later life.

## 2 Sexual dysfunction due to diabetes

Shillitoe (1988) mentions that the prevalence figures for diabetes vary as much as five to tenfold between studies, but over the age of 40 years perhaps 5–10% of the population are affected. In the study of people over 50 years by Brecher (1984), 6% of the men said that they suffered from diabetes. According to Jarrett (1986), of those suffering from the disorder, about 75% have type II diabetes mellitus with an onset in or after the fifth decade of life. It is not uncommon, therefore, for doctors to have quite a number of diabetic cases among their older patients, and some of these will be suffering from various degrees of sexual dysfunction. Various writers urge that doctors should actively seek information about this matter. Long (in Barber et al., 1989a) states that when patients are 'allowed' to volunteer information about their sex-lives, about 7% will state that they have some problem, but when information is deliberately sought, about twice that percentage will admit to problems. Estimates of the prevalence of impotence among diabetic men vary between 20% and 60% (Lehman and Jacobs, 1983). It is urged that psychological as well as physiological factors are involved in such cases of impotence (Anderson and Wolf, 1986; Fairburn *et al.*, 1982), but for older patients the physiological factors are undoubtedly the more important, psychosexual counselling having little therapeutic value (McCulloch *et al.*, 1986). However, not all diabetic sufferers are impotent. In the Brecher sample mentioned above, of the 136 diabetic men, 80% reported themselves as 'sexually active', as compared with 94% of the non-diabetic men. Butler and Lewis (1988) state that 'Most cases of diabetic-produced impotence are reversible'; their case is that the condition is often poorly controlled, and that proper regulation will often improve potency.

## 3 Vascular degeneration

Impairment of the blood supply is a recognized cause of impotency. Erectile inadequacy may be caused either by an inadequate volume and pressure of blood flowing into the cavernous bodies of the penis, or if there is too high a rate of venous drainage (Ebbhoj and Wagner, 1979; Michal, 1982). Either or both of these disabilities may be the result of abnormal processes in ageing, and are associated with conditions such as hypertension, atherosclerotic degeneration, ischemic heart disease and claudication (muscular pain on exertion due to impaired blood supply). Vascular surgery is sometimes undertaken (Michal, 1978) as a remedy for vascular degeneration, but seldom with older men. The oldest man in Michal's sample was aged 55.

An interesting aspect of vascular abnormality is the 'steal syndrome', as described by Wagner and Mitz (1981). This condition is often mistaken for psychogenic impotence: the man achieves a tolerable erection, but when he moves and tries to copulate, the extra blood required by the muscular activity reduces the arterial flow to the penis and the erection sags.

## 4 Decline in the level of androgens

Spark *et al.* (1980) studied a series of male patients, a number of whom had been considered to be impotent because of psychogenic factors, and found that 35% had abnormal hormonal levels. In another series of patients attending an outpatient clinic with the problem of erection inadequacy, 29% were considered to be suffering from the effects of hormonal factors (Slag *et al.*, 1983). The hormone testosterone is largely responsible for the maintenance of the sex drive, and although the level in the bloodstream is normally high enough to permit sexual activity throughout the whole of a man's life, it does drop with age, and such a lowered level may contribute to impotence. According to Vermeulen (1979) elderly men who remain sexually active have higher levels of circulating testosterone than those who are inactive, but it is difficult to separate cause from effect. Comfort (1980) points out that 'The role of androgen in the sexual cycle is not known. It is at least as likely that high levels result from, rather than cause, sexual arousal' (p. 887). Davidson *et al.* (1983) attribute the lessening of sexual interest and activity with ageing to the reduction in circulating testosterone, and although degenerative endocrine diseases are not common, they are a possible cause of sexual dysfunction in later life, and since many disturbances of the hormonal system can be treated, it is important that this possibility should be considered when differential diagnosis is attempted and programmes of therapy initiated.

Riley (1988) points out that some elderly men have had an enforced break in their sexual lives for a period (e.g. through widowhood) and then when they have the opportunity of renewing their sex-lives, as on remarriage, they find that they are impotent. Such men have plasma testosterone levels in the lower quartile of the normal range. It appears, therefore, that continued sexual activity helps to maintain the proper functioning of the hormonal system, and a long period of abstinence may cause degeneration. In such cases hormone replacement therapy until the proper physiological balance is restored seems indicated. Friedman *et al.* (1986) question the value of endocrine screening for impotent men, and state that in less than 2% of cases of erectile dysfunction endocrine factors are implicated, but this question is obviously highly related to the age of the patients. Because of the previously held erroneous stereotype of the sexless older male, little research has been done on older people. There is some evidence (Riley 1989) that with ageing the testes slowly decline in their androgen-producing function. The relevant tissue, the Leydig cells, ceases to respond to the gonadotrophin stimulation, and indeed the actual number of the cells begins to decrease after the age of 50 (Neaves and Johnson, 1984), so we have a slow process in the male somewhat similar to the rapid process in the female when the ovaries cease to secrete the female hormones and the menopause occurs. However, for most men there is an adequate though reduced level of testosterone which permits sexual activity for the whole of their lives.

## 5 Generalized metabolic disturbance

The generalized metabolic disturbances that become more frequent with age tend to suppress the sexual drive and capability. Conditions such as chronic renal failure have the specific effect of lowering sexual drive, and strangely, while renal dialysis may re-awaken sexual interest, it tends to abolish sexual function (Bancroft, 1982). It is generally accepted that decline in physical health has a de-sexualizing effect in ageing people (Martin, 1977), but Brecher (1984) reveals some curious facts concerning his large study of people over 50 years. He studied seven specific health impairments in relation to their impact on sexual behaviour, and reports:

> Even the largest of these impacts of health on sexuality, however, is smaller than the impact of aging on sexuality. . . . Remarkably large proportions, both men and women, report being sexually active, engaging in sex at least once a week, and with high enjoyment of sex – despite only fair or poor health, and despite the seven adverse health factors here reviewed (Brecher, 1984, p. 286).

## 6 Sexual problems following prostatectomy

As the physiology of the ageing male body sometimes makes the operation of prostatectomy necessary, many men fear that they will lose their sexual capacity because of this. In fact, three methods of performing this operation, transuretheral, suprapubic and retropubic prostatectomy, have little effect on erectile capacity, although there is experimentally based evidence that it does have some effect on nocturnal erections (Madorsky, 1976). However, the layman's fears about the effects of the operation may produce a psychogenic impotence, and it is therefore necessary to give preoperative counselling, assuring the patient that after recovery from the operation he will be little affected. It is necessary to explain that in one particular he may be affected, and that is that there may be some change in the process of ejaculation. Retrograde ejaculation, that is, the semen being forced into the bladder, may take place. However, as men over the age of 60 are seldom concerned about the procreative aspects of sexual intercourse, this is not likely to be a serious problem.

The radical perineal operation, which is generally performed in cases of prostatic carcinoma, is likely to be followed by complete erectile failure, partly because it causes incidental damage to neural tissue, and patients should be counselled about this in advance.

## 7 Ejaculatory dysfunctions

The problems outlined above under six headings have all dealt with erectile inadequacy, but we should also consider the question of ejaculatory dysfunction which may be brought about by medically prescribed drugs, diabetes, and other factors that are increasingly encountered as we age. Typically, trouble with ejaculation (especially premature ejaculation) is the problem of the younger man, but erectile incompetence is the problem of the older. In the studies of young men and those in early middle age by Catalan et al. (1981) and Frank et al. (1978), although there was a much greater incidence of sexual problems in the latter study, the ratio of premature ejaculation to erectile incompetence was about 2:1 in both. In so far as Brecher (1984) cites relevant figures for men in their 50s, 60s and 70+, the position appears to be reversed in older men.

The relationship between erectile and ejaculatory dysfunction in older men is not at all clear. Comfort (1980) states:

It is important to recognize that human sexual function, especially in the male, is *highly idiosyncratic*, both in the interrelation of the erectile function and ejaculatory functions, and the response of these functions to drugs. Medication which produces impotence in one individual may produce non-ejaculation or anterograde ejaculation in another, and be without sexual effects on a third, as had been documented in the case of thioridazine (Comfort, 1980, p. 886).

Kothari (1984) objects to the common term 'ejaculatory dys-function' because it 'compounds confusion and propagates the erroneous belief that ejaculation and orgasm in men are one and the same.' He makes the point, that is highly relevant to counsel-ling older men, that we should be primarily concerned with the erotic component of making love rather than when and where semen is discharged. He proposes that we should consider a terminology of 'early orgasmic response', 'delayed orgasmic response', 'absent orgasmic response', and 'incomplete orgasmic response'. This makes good sense when discussing the sexual satisfaction of the older man and his partner. Young men (and to a lesser extent young women) tend to conceive of lovemaking as a run-up to the important event of seminal ejaculation. Older men have to learn that there is a lot more to lovemaking than that, and when they have realized that the criteria by which they judged their sexual performance in their younger years are no longer appropriate, they can adapt to a sex-life that is somewhat different but none the less satisfying to both partners. This point will be discussed further later in this book.


## ADVICE AND THERAPY FOR OLDER MEN

Most counselling for ageing men need not be very elaborate. What they chiefly need is to be given the basic facts about the processes of normal ageing, as outlined above, and reassured that although their sexual capacity with alter with ageing, they need not expect to lose their masculinity as a matter of course. It may be necessary to counter several myths about male sexuality that are current, and to get men to talk about what they believe will happen with ageing. Many of those who are now in the genera-tions over the age of 60 are likely to believe in some of the myths about male sexuality, and some myths about women, that were current in the earlier part of this century, and even received some

**Table 1.5** Myths about sexuality and ageing

1. Intercourse and emission of semen are debilitating and will tend to hasten old age and death.
2. One's sex life can be prolonged by abstinence in earlier years and inactivity in later years.
3. Masturbation is a childish activity that is put aside with one reaches adulthood, and is carried out by older persons only if they are seriously disturbed.
4. Coital satisfaction decreases considerably after the menopause.
5. Older men are particularly subject to sexual deviations, for example, exhibitionism and child molesting.
6. Older women who still enjoy sex were probably nymphomaniacs when they were younger.
7. Most older men lose their ability and desire to have sex.
8. Sexual ability and performance remain the same throughout life.
9. If older individuals go without sex for several years, they will not be able to have sex at a future time.
10. Older people with chronic illness or physical disabilities should cease sex activity completely.

Croft, L.H. (1982) *Sexuality in Later Life* Appendix B, John Wright, Boston. Reprinted by permission.

medical backing. Croft (1981) gives a list of myths about sexuality and ageing that are still current, as shown in Table 1.5.

It is worth while to initiate discussion of each of these myths, as some men may be diffident about expressing the fears that worry them, and unwilling to admit the extent of their ignorance. It may be noted that while most of the myths listed imply that sexuality simply disappears in the later years, No. 8, which states that 'Sexual ability and performance remain the same throughout life' is mischievous for the older man as it implies that if he cannot perform as he used to in his youth, there is something wrong with him. All men have a failure of potency on a few occasions of attempted intercourse, and while this is so at all ages due to a variety of circumstances, it becomes increasingly likely as they get older. The danger is that one or two incidents of failed potency in an ageing man may convince him that he is now 'impotent' and that he may therefore withdraw from all attempts at lovemaking for fear of the 'humiliation' of such an experience. Thus a condition of performance anxiety may develop in relation to sex, and he becomes impotent for psychogenic reasons while he is perfectly well able to perform physiologically, although less regularly than when he was younger. In some such cases, Cole

21

(1985) uses surrogate sex partners, a practice that was pioneered by Masters and Johnson (1970). These surrogates are women who are skilled at putting a man at his ease and restoring his confidence in his ability to have normal intercourse. Once confidence is restored, the patient may find that he can return to making love normally with his wife or regular sex partner.

## Towards a new concept of lovemaking

The use of surrogate therapy is obviously an expensive and elaborate form of therapy, and will be quite unacceptable to some men for moral and other reasons. It is of limited help to those men whose capacity really is impaired to some degree by physiological conditions such as those described earlier in this chapter. Many sex therapists are now coming to take a new look at the whole emotional and physical processes we refer to as lovemaking, and to question whether the act of intercourse, culminating in a seminal ejaculation, is not given too much importance. They point out that what is really important for both partners is the giving and receiving of mutual affection and pleasure, and this can be achieved by a great variety of techniques, extending over whatever period of time they wish. McCarthy (1977) points out that our existing terminology of sexuality tends to underrate the importance of experiencing emotional gratification and the associated pleasure, and overrates the achievement of a goal.

Historically, as the procreation of children has been the prime biological object of sexuality, the male's act of the implantation of seed has acquired great symbolic importance, and the symbol is still important even when sex is engaged in for recreational purposes. In the later years of life, however, lovemaking is the vehicle maintaining the pair-bond, and the affirmation of love between two people. Touching, caressing and shared delight assume a greater importance in the later years of life, and that is why in the research studies of the opinions of older people (Brecher, 1984; Starr and Weiner, 1981) so many people say that sex is now 'better' than when they were younger, although the frequency of intercourse is less.

The whole question of the sex education suitable for older people will be deferred for further discussion in Chapter 8.

## Androgen therapy for ageing men

As described earlier in this chapter, there is a decline in the level of plasma testosterone with ageing, and with some men the level is so low that the sexual drive disappears and they become generally sexually inadequate. Riley (1989) says that such men 'may gain great benefit from a short course of androgen supplementation', but warns that 'Erectile dysfunction in men with normal plasma testosterone levels is not an indication for androgen therapy, except where the erectile dysfunction is secondary to loss of sexual desire'. This would imply that the hormonal supplementation serves as a boost to the man's sexual drive, and once he begins an active sex life the situation will right itself. As sexual dysfunction in the male is multifactorial, such medication should be accompanied by measures of counselling and behavioural therapy by specialists where feasible. It used to be thought that about 90% of cases of erectile dysfunction were psychogenic, but later researchers put more emphasis on organic factors, Melman *et al.* (1984) suggesting that about 70% of cases are organic. Friedman (1988) suggests that the pendulum has swung too far in the attribution of organic causes, but as one goes up the age scale, obviously organic factors will become more important.

One gets the impression that at present the issue of androgen therapy for men is rather controversial, and those using it are proceeding with caution.

## Artificial means of attaining erection

There are a number of techniques for obtaining erection which do not depend on overcoming inhibiting emotional factors or on strengthening the sexual drive. Virag (1982) demonstrated that the injection of papaverine, an opium derivative, into the intercavernous spaces of the penis would be vasoactive to the extent that an erection would occur, and Brindley (1986) published a report of its clinical use. It is estimated that over 10,000 patients in the USA have now been treated by this form of therapy. How far a man will enjoy intercourse with a penis rendered erect by this means will depend on a number of factors. However, he may be able to satisfy his partner, and most importantly, if the lack of proper function has resulted from performance anxiety and other psychogenic causes, the fact of performing normally on a number of occasions may give the man such a boost to his confidence that proper function will return, and the treatment will not be necessary on future occasions.

This treatment has now been commercialized, and private clinics offering the service advertise in the newspapers. The treatment is not without its hazards, the principal of which is that it may cause priapism, a dangerous condition in which the penis remains painfully erect for a very long time, and medical intervention is necessary if resolution does not occur after 12 hours. Doctors using this treatment therefore have to be available to deal with any complications around the clock.

The injection of papaverine is not only a form of treatment, but it has its use in the diagnosis of the aetiology of penile dysfunction – whether it is primarily psychogenic, neurogenic, or vasculogenic, – different responses to the drug indicating the nature of the disorder. Different forms of therapy can be initiated when the exact nature of the dysfunction has been determined. Diagnosis is a highly specialized matter, and Guirguis (1989) gives details, and indicates where medical practitioners can obtain training in the techniques of diagnosis and treatment.

Quite recently Jeremy and Mikhailidis (1989) have published details of their ongoing research into another agent, prostacyclin, which does not have the disadvantage of papaverine carrying the risk of long-continued erection that may lead to priapism. Virag et al. (1987) claim that the beneficial effects of prostacyclin can last for months. It will be of great interest to see how this research proceeds, and whether an agent can be developed that will be effective when administered via an oral route. It must be stressed that such agents can be of little use when the dysfunction is caused by serious impairment of the arterial supply to the penis, as with atherosclerotic lesions, or when there is denervation of the penis, as in advanced cases of diabetic neuropathy.

Penile implants should also be mentioned among the artificial means of inducing or simulating erections. This is a very old idea, and there are a wide variety of devices, some of them simple, rigid supports, and some complex devices whereby a tube in the penis can be inflated to make the organ partly stiff. How effective these devices are depends very much on the attitude of the man concerned. The fact that some men are prepared to have operations to have them implanted must mean that they are perceived as valuable by some people and may serve as a confidence-boosting device.

## Aphrodisiac drugs

The search for substances that will increase sexual desire in both sexes and boost sexual performance is very ancient, and is responsible for a great deal of folk-lore. Some of the traditional preparations, such as cantharides, are definitely dangerous. It cannot be stated definitely that no drug under any circumstances can enhance sexual desire and/or performance, but most of the favourable reports of their use has undoubtedly been due to the placebo effect. There is, however one drug, yohimbine, an indole alkaloid, which has traditionally been used as an aphrodisiac, and which is currently the subject of renewed attention. Morales *et al.* (1981) used it in a small study with impotent men, and the favourable results prompted them to try it in a controlled trial compared with a placebo (Morales *et al.*, 1984). Preliminary results have been encouraging, but we must await the results of further research on a larger scale.

## REFERENCES

Anderson, B.J. and Wolf, F.M. (1986) Chronic physical illness and sexual behavior: psychological issues, *J. Consult. Clin. Psychol.*, 54, 168–175.
Bancroft, J. (1983) *Human Sexuality and Its Problems*, Churchill Livingstone, Edinburgh.
Barber, E.D., Butler, R.N., Lewis, M., Long, J. and Whitehead, E.D. (1989a) Sexual problems in the elderly. I. The use and abuse of medications, *Geriatrics*, 44, 61–71.
Brecher, E.M. (1984) *Love, Sex, and Aging: A Consumer Union Report*, Little, Brown & Co., Boston.
Bretschneider, J.G. and McCoy, N.L. (1988) Sexual interest and behaviour in healthy 80 to 102 year olds, *Arch. Sex. Behav.*, 17, 109–129.
Brindley, G.S. (1986) Maintenance treatment of erectile impotency by cavernosal unstriated muscle relaxant injection, *Br. J. Psychiat.*, 149, 210–215.
Butler, R.N. and Lewis, M.I. (1988) *Love and Sex After 60*, Harper & Row, New York.

Catalan, J., Bradley, M., Gallway, J. and Horton, K. (1981) Sexual dysfunction and psychiatric morbidity in patients attending a clinic for sexually transmitted diseases, *Br. J. Psychiat.*, 138, 292–296.

Cole, M. (1988) Sex therapy for individuals, in Cole, M. and Dryden, W. (eds) *Sex Therapy in Britain*, pp. 272–299, Open University Press, Milton Keynes.

Comfort, A. (1979) *The Biology of Senescence*, 3rd edn, Elsevier, New York.

Comfort, A. (1980) Sexuality in later life, in Birren, J.E. and Sloane, R.L. (eds) *Handbook of Mental Health and Aging*, Prentice Hall, Englewood Cliffs, N.J.

Comfort, A. (1990) *A Good Age*, Pan Books, London.

Cooper, G.F. (1988) The psychological methods of sex therapy, in Cole, M. and Dryden, W. (eds) *Sex Therapy in Britain*, pp. 127–164, Open University Press, Milton Keynes.

Croft, L.H. (1982) *Sexuality in the Later Years*, John Wright, Boston.

Davidson, J.M., Chen, J.J., Crapo, L., Gray, D.G., Greenleaf, W.J. and Catana, J.A. (1983) Hormonal changes and sexual function in aging men, *J. Clin. Endocrin. Metabol.*, 57, 71–77.

Dunn, M.E. and Trost, J.E. (1989) Male multiple orgasms: a descriptive study, *Archiv. Sex. Behav.*, 18, 377–387.

Ebbhoj, J. and Wagner, G. (1979) Insufficient penile erection due to abnormal drainage of the cavernous bodies, *Urology*, 13, 507–510.

Ellis, H. (1933), *The Psychology of Sex: A Manual for Students*, W. Heinemann, London.

Fairburn, C.G., Wu, F.C.W. and McCulloch, D.K. (1982) The clinical features of diabetic impotence: a preliminary study, *Br. J. Psychiat.*, 140, 447–452.

Finkle, A.L., Moyers, T.G., Tobenkin, E. and Karg, S.J. (1959) Sexual potency in aging males, I. Frequency of coitus among clinic patients, *J. Am. Med. Ass.*, 196, 139.

Fisher, C., Cohen, H.D., Schiari, R.C. *et al.* (1983) Patterns of female sexual arousal during sleep and waking: vaginal thermo-conductance studies. *Arch. Sex. Behav.*, 12, 97–122.

Frank, E., Anderson, C. and Rubinstein, D. (1978), Frequency of sexual dysfunction in 'normal' couples, *New Eng. J. Med.*, 299, 111–115.

Freidman, D. (1988) Assessing the basis of sexual dysfunction: diagnostic procedures, in Cole, M. and Dryden, W. (eds) *Sex Therapy in Britain*, pp. 105–124, Open University Press, Milton Keynes.

Freidman, D., Clare, A.W., Rees, L.H. and Grossman, A. (1986) Should impotent males who have no clinical evidence of hypogonadism have routine endocrine screening? *The Lancet*, i, 1041.

George, L.K. and Weiler, S.J. (1981) Sexuality in middle and late life: the effects of age, cohort and gender, *Arch. Gen. Psychiat.*, 38, 919–923.

Guirguis, W.R. (1989) The use and abuse of intercavernous injection of vasoactive drugs, *Br. J. Sex. Med.*, 16, 9–11.

Heath, R.G. (1972) Pleasure and brain activity in man, *J. Nerv. Ment. Dis.*, 154, 3–18.

Jarrett, R.J. (1986) *Diabetes Mellitus*, Croom Helm, London.

Jeremy, J.Y. and Mikhailidis, D.P. (1989) Prostanoids and impotence, *Br. J. Sex. Med.*, 16, 411–413.

Kaplan, S. (1974) *The New Sex Therapy*, Bruner/Mazel, New York.

Kinsey, A.C., Pomeroy, W.B. and Martin, C.D. (1948) *Sexual Behavior in the Human Male*, W.B. Saunders & Co., New York.

Kothari, P. (1984) Ejaculatory dysfunctions – a new dimension. *Br. J. Sex. Med.*, 11, 205–209.

Lehman, T.P. and Jacobs, J.A. (1983) Etiology of diabetic impotence, *J. Urol.*, 129, 291–294.

McCarthy, B.W. (1977) *What You Don't Know About Male Sexuality*, T.Y. Crowell, New York.

McCulloch, D.K., Hosking, D.J. and Tobert, A. (1986) A pragmatic approach to sexual dysfunction in diabetic men: psychosexual counselling, *Diabetic Med.*, 3, 485–489.

Madorsky, I.L., Ashamalla, M.J., Schussler, I., Lyons, H.R. and Miller, G.H. Jnr. (1976) Prostatectomy impotence, *J. Urol.*, 115, 401–403.

Martin, C. (1977) Sexual activity in the aging male, in Money, J. and Musaph, H. (eds) *Handbook of Sexology*, Excerpta Medica, Amsterdam.

Masters, W.H. and Johnson, V.E. (1966) *Human Sexual Response*, Little, Brown & Co, Boston.

Masters, W.H. and Johnson, V.E. (1970) *Human Sexual Inadequacy*, J.A. Churchill, London.

Melman, A., Kaplan, D. and Redfield, J. (1984) Evaluation of the first 70 patients in the Center for Male Sexual Dysfunction of Beth Israel Medical Center, *J. Urol.*, 131, 53–55.

Michal, V. (1982) Arterial disease as a cause of impotence, *Clinics in Endocrinol. Metabol.*, 2, 725–748.

Mikhailidis, D.P., Jeremy, J.Y., Barradas, M.A., Green, N. and Dandona, P. (1983) Effect of ethanol on vascular prostacyclin (prostaglandin I) synthesis, platelet aggregation, and platelet thromboxane release, *Br. Med. J.*, 287, 1495–1498.

Morales, A., Surridge, D.H. and Marshall, P.G. (1981) Yohimbine for treatment of impotence in diabetes, *New Eng. J. Med.*, 305, 1221.

Morales, A., Condra, M., Surridge, D.S.H., Fennemore, J. and Owen, J.A. (1984) The effects of yohimbine in the treatment of impotence: results of a controlled trial, *Am. Urolog. Assoc. Meeting Abstracts*, A.391.

Neaves, W.B. and Johnson, L. (1984) Age-related changes in numbers of insterstitial cells in the human testis: evidence bearing on the fate of Leydig cells lost with increasing age, *17th Annual Meeting of the Society for the Study of Reproduction, Laramie*, Abstract 100.

Pfeiffer, E., Verwoerdt, A. and Davis, G.C. (1972) Sexual behavior in middle life, *Am. J. Psychiat.*, 128, 1267.

Riley, A.J. (1988) The endocrinology of sexual function and dysfunction, in Cole, M. and Dryden, W. (eds) *Sex Therapy in Britain*, pp. 69–90, Open University Press, Milton Keynes.

Riley A.J. (1989) Male sexual dysfunction, *Br. J. Sex. Med.*, 16, 271–273.

Robbins, M.B. and Jensen, G.D. (1978) Multiple orgasm in males, *J.*

*Sex. Res.*, 14, 21–26.

Shillitoe, R.W. (1988) *Psychology and Diabetes*, Chapman & Hall, London.

Slag, M.F., Morley, J.E., Elson, M.K. *et al.* (1983) Impotence in medical clinic outpatients, *J. Am. Med. Ass.*, 249, 1736–1740.

Spark, R.F., White, R.A. and Connolly, P.B. (1980) Impotence is not always psychogenic: new insights into hypothalamic-pituitary-gonadal dysfunction, *J. Am. Med. Ass.*, 243, 750–755.

Starr, B.D. (1985) Sexuality and aging, *Ann. Rev. Gerontol.*, 5, 97–126.

Starr, B.D. and Weiner, M.B. (1981) *The Starr-Weiner Report on Sex and Sexuality in the Mature Years*, McGraw Hill, New York.

Vermeulen, A. (1979) Decline in sexual activity in aging men: correlation with sex hormone levels and testicular changes. *J. Biosocial Sci.*, (Suppl.) 6, 5–18.

Virag, R. (1982) Intercavernous injection of papaverine for erectile failure, *The Lancet*, 2, 939.

Virag, R. and Adaikan, P.G. (1987) Effects of prostaglandin E1 on penile erection and erectile failure, *J. Urol.*, 137, 1010.

Wagner, G. and Mitz, P. (1981) Arteriosclerosis and erectile failure, in Wagner, G. and Green, R. (eds) *Impotence: Physiological Psychological, Surgical Diagnosis and Treatment*, p. 63–72, Plenum Press, New York.

# 2

# The physiology of age-related changes in sexual capacity and experience: a plan for therapy. II Women

As in the case of men, it will be necessary first to outline the facts about the experience and behaviour of women in their later years with regard to their emotional and sexual lives, then to describe the normal physiological changes that accompany ageing. The abnormalities of function that require the attention of professional health-care workers are described, and finally the question of counselling and therapy is discussed.

## THE NORMAL SEXUAL BEHAVIOUR AND EXPERIENCE OF OLDER WOMEN

All that must be said about women in this context must be considered against a social background of a steady increase in the numerical discrepancy between the two sexes as they age. Many women are debarred from heterosexual experience in their later lives because there are just not enough male partners. This matter will be fully discussed in Chapter 6.

Kinsey's second report, *Sexual Behavior in the Human Female* (Kinsey *et al.*, 1953) concerned relatively few older people, as has already been noted, and his tables stop at age 65. However, it covers the important years around the menopause, and the decade following it, and contains much valuable data. On the basis of his researches he and his colleagues made the following important observation:

> The incidences of responding males, and the frequencies of response to the point of orgasm reach their peak within three to four years after the onset of adolescence. On the other hand, the maximum incidences of sexually responding females

are not approached until some time in the late twenties and in the thirties.

The frequencies of sexual response in the male begin to decline after the late teens or early twenties, and drop steadily into old age. On the other hand . . . among females the median frequencies of those sexual activities that are not dependent upon the male's initiation of socio-sexual contacts [e.g., masturbation] remain more or less constant from the late teens into the fifties and sixties (Kinsey *et al.*, 1953, pp. 714–715).

Kinsey's data, inadequate though they are as regards the number of older people, showed a slight decline in the sexual activity of women in the fifties and early sixties, but a decline in frequency does not mean a cessation. Newman and Nichols (1960), who studied men and women between the ages of 60 and 93 years, found that if women remained healthy they continued to be sexually active for the whole of their lives. The latter finding was confirmed by Masters and Johnson (1966) (albeit basing their observations about older women on only 56 aged 51–78 years) who stated that 'there is no time limit drawn by the advancing years to female sexuality' (p. 247). However, it is difficult to decide just what criteria of 'sexual activity' we are to use. If a woman reports that she has fairly frequent intercourse with her husband, that may mean that she actively desires it and is often the initiator, or that she merely tolerates it to please her husband although she has no active sex drive. We have already noted that in the older age-groups frequency of intercourse for a woman is no real guide as to her sexual drive, for as we go up the age gradient there are more and more women without male partners.

Kinsey took the frequency of self-masturbation (with or without intercourse in addition) as an indicator of the strength of the sex drive, and if we consider this as valid, the data produced by Starr and Weiner (1981) are of relevance. They asked their respondents (n = 443) the question 'Do you masturbate?': for men, 52.6% of the 60–69 age group, and 32.7% of those 70+ replied 'Yes', a drop of nearly 20% with ageing. For women there was no such significant drop with age, the relevant percentages being 47.1% and 46.8%. Somewhat similar figures are given by Brecher (1984) who also asked about masturbation in his questionnaire, and found that the drop in frequency was far more pronounced in men than in women. Starr and Weiner's data are also of interest in that they show that although the difference in the incidence of female masturbation is in the expected direction, there is not a great deal of difference between the married, widowed, divorced and single women, indicating that it is not simply a practice engendered by sexual privation. Catania and White (1982) investigated the matter, and concluded that masturbation was one way in which ageing people maintained their sexual identity and confirmed their continued sexuality in the face of society's dismissive stereotype of them as being asexual.

Croft (1982) observes that 'Research in the area of aged female sexuality is particularly ambiguous and contradictory. There is slightly more agreement about aged male sexuality from a physiological standpoint' (p. 10). This is commented on by a number of writers. For instance in Table 1.1 the data of Pfeiffer *et al.* (1972) are given, showing that, in their sample, when sexual relations in marriage were terminated it was generally due to the incapacity of the husband. This view of the decline of sexual interest or activity in older married women being largely due to illness or lowered capacity and interest on the part of the husband, is also advanced by White (1982) on the basis of his research. However, other researchers have found the contrary effect in the samples they have studied (e.g. Wasow and Loeb, 1975; Hegeler and Mortensen, 1978), and one has to consider very carefully the nature of each particular study, and the circumstances under which questions were asked, in order to gain some insight into why the data appear as they do. We are, after all, recording what men and women *say* about their behaviour and feelings, and there is certainly quite a pronounced difference between men and women, especially those brought up in the early part of this century, as to their willingness to be entirely frank with strangers about their sex-lives, however professionally respectable the researchers may be. As well as the differences between the sexes, there are the differences between the generations to be taken into account. If women in their fifties admit to a certain types of sexual activity much more frequently than women in their seventies, this difference will partly reflect the fact that the latter group may be rather more reticent about sexual practices than the former, having been brought up when social conventions were more restrictive.

Because of the relatively restricted opportunities for most sexual activities for women as compared with men, it is pertinent to distinguish between *sexual activity* and *sexual interest*. Various researchers have inquired into this matter, and in the longitudinal studies of community volunteers at Duke University, the first of which began in 1954, Verwoerdt *et al*. (1969) found that the high and moderate sexual interest of women continued to a late age, and exceeded the incidence of overt sexual activity. This finding has been confirmed by many subsequent studies.

It is instructive to study the sexual practices of older people, and society's attitudes to them, in other cultures. Winn and Newton (1982) reviewed anthropological studies of 106 cultures and found that in 84% of them women continued to be sexually active into advanced old age. In quite a number of cultures, older women were used as the sexual initiators and instructors of younger men, although there was a general tendency of older men to marry younger women, a practice that has a direct bearing or the continued fertility of older men, while the child-bearing age of women ceases in early middle age. In contrast with what has generally been assumed in advanced Western societies, there are reports from all over the world of cultures in which women become more sexually active after the menopause, and much less inhibited in their sexual behaviour than women of child-bearing age. In general, these anthropological reports strongly support the finding that women pursue an active sex-life into old age to a significantly greater degree than do men.

## The normal sexual response of the female

In Chapter 1 the normal sexual response of the male was described according to the four-phase model proposed by Masters and Johnson (1966). The female response was also described by them in terms of the same four phases, and it will be convenient to adhere to this model here.

(i) The excitement phase. In response to sexual stimulation vaginal lubrication occurs in 15–30 seconds, and this is accompanied by other changes. The vaginal barrel distends involuntarily, and erectile tissue of the pudenda, which is homologous with that in the male, is suffused with blood. The nipples also erect, and there are changes in the major and minor labia that make penetration easier.

(ii) The plateau phase. Vaginal lubrication is maintained, as are the changes effected by the engorgement of the erectile tissue.

(iii) The orgasmic phase. According to Masters and Johnson, the female orgasm is triggered by stimulation of the clitoris, either directly, or indirectly in intercourse by penile thrusting pulling on other parts of the sexual organs. The uterus contracts reflexly and rhythmically, and there are neural discharges, as in the male, that have been likened to a minor epileptic fit by Kinsey et al. (1953). In contrast to the male, there is just one stage in the orgasm. It may be noted here that not everyone agrees with Masters and Johnson about the nature of the female orgasm. According to Cole and Dryden (1988b) 'many women report quite different types of orgasm and sites of stimulation, which can be roughly divided into the 'clitoral-vulval' and the 'vaginal-uterine' (p. 8). There is indeed much evidence from later studies, as discussed by Levin (1981), that makes it apparent that the Masters and Johnson model of the female orgasm is rather over-simple.

(iv) The resolution phase. Unlike in the male, resolution occurs as a continuous process with women. Also, unlike the male, for many women there is no easily definable refractory period in which they cannot be re-aroused sexually. We owe it chiefly to researchers later than Masters and Johnson to appreciate how some women can achieve multiple orgasms, remaining in the plateau phase between such events. According to Wilson (1988) 'Multiple orgasm is possible for women because they do not ejaculate – a capacity that exists in some prepubertal boys for the same reason'.

### Normal physiological changes with ageing

To describe these changes Masters and Johnson (1966; 1970) refer to 'the older woman' (50–70 years), and 'the younger woman' (20–40 years). Why age 70 is the upper limit is because they had not studied women over that age and were therefore being cautious. That they did not believe that the sex-life of women ended at age 70 is evident from their statement that

'There are only two basic needs for regularity of sexual expression in 70–80-year-old women. These necessities are a reasonably good state of general health and an interested and interesting partner' (Masters and Johnson, 1966, p. 350). Even here they feel it necessary to specify an upper age of 80 years! In the last chapter we have cited Brecher's (1984) finding that health in later life is not so important for a satisfying sex-life as was once thought.

As with the male, the physiological changes in the sexual response of the female will be considered in terms of the postulated four phases.

(i) Excitement phase. In contrast with the younger woman who experiences vagina lubrication within 15–30 seconds, the older woman may not react thus until after about five minutes of sexual stimulation. As before, the vaginal barrel distends involuntarily, but the reaction happens more slowly and less extensively in the older woman, and the lining to the vagina has become much thinner. This varies very much with individual women, and is related to the relative level of the sex steroids available after the menopause.

(ii) Plateau phase. The changes in the labia and in the clitoris that are apparent in the plateau phase are less obvious in the older woman, there being some minor anatomical changes in the erected clitoris similar to those in the male penis, but Masters and Johnson (1970) comment, 'there is no objective evidence to date to suggest that there is any appreciable loss in sensate focus'.

(iii) Orgasmic phase. This phase is shortened in the older woman, and the natural uterine contraction pattern may follow two alternative reaction pathways. The first is like that of the younger woman, but with fewer reflex contractions on orgasm, and the second is a spastic rather than a rhythmic contraction, and the spasm of the uterus may last as long as a minute. Abnormally, this spasm may be perceived as painful, and again, it reflects the level of sex steroids.

(iv) Resolution phase. This occurs more rapidly in the older woman. No reliable data are available as to there being any change in the capacity for experiencing multiple orgasms with ageing.

Age-related changes have been described in terms of Masters and Johnson's four-phase model for the sake of convenience, but it should be noted that later writers have criticized this model, and the interpretation that was put on the events described. It seems likely that the older people presenting at Masters and Johnson's clinic were mostly suffering from various sorts of disability, and they had not a wide enough experience of normally functioning older men and women.

Kaplan (1974) offers a three-stage model of *sexual desire, excitement* and *orgasm*, and Cooper (1988) offers a four-stage model of *desire, arousal, orgasm* and *resolution*. However, these different ways of considering the sexual cycle do not alter materially the account given by Masters and Johnson, or the changes that they record as taking place with ageing. The importance of considering the phase of desire is that one can discuss 'disorders of desire' as an emotional disorder separate from the physiological concomitants of arousal, a question that is particularly relevant to women.

Such are the basic facts about the normal age-related physiological changes in the sexual response of females. In general, women alter less than men physiologically with ageing, except for the all-important factor of the menopause which affects the level of the sex steroids that are available, and this varies very greatly between individuals, and is fortunately susceptible to treatment by hormone replacement therapy. The question of the menopause will be dealt with in a separate section.

### The Menopause

There is now an enormous literature devoted to research into the menopause, and an international journal, *Maturitas*, devoted to such research. With the growing body of research literature it has become evident that some of what was previously regarded as fact is more questionable now, because the great inter-individual variation in menopausal patterns has come into increasing prominence. While younger and uninformed women regard the coming menopause rather with apprehension and dread, many post-menopausal women express considerable satisfaction because they no longer have to be concerned with contraception and the whole business of having periods (Neugarten *et al.*, 1968). That sexual activity is much more satisfactory for the average post-menopausal woman than for the average man over 60, was strikingly revealed in the Starr-Weiner Report (Starr and Weiner,

**Table 2.1** Responses to the question 'How does sex feel now compared with when you were younger?' put to people over 60 years.

| Response | Men | | Women | |
|---|---|---|---|---|
| | N | % | N | % |
| 'Better' | 74 | 27.1 | 181 | 41.0 |
| 'The same' | 102 | 37.4 | 175 | 39.7 |
| 'Worse' | 97 | 35.5 | 85 | 19.3 |
| Total | 273 | | 441 | |

Figures derived from Starr, B.D. and Weiner, M.B. (1981) *The Starr–Weiner Report on Sex and Sexuality in the Mature Years*, McGraw Hill, New York.

1981). The 441 women and 273 men who replied to the question 'How does sex feel now compared with when you were younger?' gave responses as shown in Table 2.1.

It should be remembered that the population responding to this question was self-selected out of a larger pool of people approached, and therefore probably happier about their sex-lives than the general population at large. However, that only 19.3% of post-menopausal women replied that sex was 'worse' as compared with 35.5% of men, indicates that the menopause is less of a handicap to women than the ordinary process of ageing is to men. Perhaps surprisingly, as many as 41.0% of women found it 'better' compared with 27.1% of men. The study did not reveal, of course, how many of these satisfied women were having the benefit of hormone replacement therapy.

Dalton (1978) gives an average age for the menopause as 48 years, with a normal range of 45–55 years, for British women, and such an estimate is generally accepted. Kaufert *et al.* (1987) state that 'Menopause itself is defined as a woman's last menses, and a woman is postmenopausal if she says that she has not menstruated within the past 12 months' (p. 218). Although the terms 'male menopause' and 'male climacteric' are sometimes encountered in the literature (e.g. Utian, 1978), they have no real status in scientific studies as there is no process of relatively sudden and irreversible hormonal change in men comparable with what naturally occurs in women.

The changes in the woman are mainly due to the reduction in the level of oestrogen in the system. The lower level of hormones affects those tissues which contain oestrogen receptors (Taylor, 1974) such as in the breast, the uterus, ovaries, fallopian tubes, vagina, vulva and the terminal portion of the urethra. A degree of atrophy may occur in these organs post-menstrually in proportion with the oestrogen lack, and such atrophy is associated with lower levels of sexual drive and activity. The physiological changes naturally interact with emotional factors related to the individual woman's perception of herself, and possible changes in her relationship with her sexual partner. There is even some slight evidence that the sexual attraction between partners is altered by changes in the pheromones emitted by the woman in the postmenopausal period (Morris and Udry, 1975), and Riley (1988) comments 'Clinical experience has shown that some men experience improved sexual functioning when their postmenopausal partners receive oestrogen replacement therapy. Whether this is a pheromonal effect remains to be shown' (p. 78).

As well as changes in the sexual organs, alterations in the hormonal system produce such unwelcome phenomena as hot flushes and a tendency to osteoporosis. However, in this chapter we shall deal only with the physiological changes that have a direct bearing on changes in female sexual functioning due to the menopause. Modern writers tend to discount the older idea that the menopause brings about profound changes in women's emotional stability, as it is now realized that any such changes are brought about by factors in the individual's general psycho-social circumstances, including her sex life. Much of what has been written about the decline of sexual interest and activity in postmenopausal women is, as noted earlier, somewhat contradictory, different research studies showing inconsistent results that are difficult to interpret. We are reminded again and again that such data must be considered in the light of what is happening to the women's ageing sexual partners. When dealing with populations that are predominantly middle-class, as in the Starr-Weiner study mentioned above, we should also consider that nowadays a percentage are probably enjoying the benefits of hormone replacement supplements. The women who admit to a marked decrease of sexual interest and activity are often those in the lowest socio-economic class (Jaszmann, 1973; Van Keep and Kellerhals, 1974), and such women are less prone to get their doctors to prescribe hormone supplements, being more content to suffer in silence without actively seeking a remedy.

## ABNORMAL DISABILITIES IN THE SEXUAL FUNCTION OF AGEING WOMEN

### 1 Painful intercourse

Painful intercourse (dyspareunia) in the post-menopausal woman is generally due to less efficient vaginal lubrication, and the thinning of the vaginal epithelium, these being the result of oestrogen deficiency. Urinary discomfort following intercourse can also result from the impaired cushioning effect of the thinner vaginal wall. Masters and Johnson (1970) also observed that dyspareunia is less likely to occur in the post-menopausal woman is she has had regular and frequent sexual intercourse, but if this is generally the case, the meaning is not clear. It might be that such a woman has had a high level of oestrogen in the first place, and her frequent sexual activity was a consequence of this, or it might be that such activity promotes and sustains the proper functioning of the hormonal system.

Partial atrophy of the vagina and labia, and insufficient lubrication, will naturally cause some discomfort on intercourse, and this will discourage a woman from full participation in the act. Hormone replacement therapy will halt that process of atrophy and increase vaginal lubrication, but it is not clear whether the restoration of a proper hormone level will in itself actually increase sexual interest and desire, or whether such increase is a secondary effect of more enjoyable experience.

Even if the mechanics of the system are in perfect working order potentially, if psychological factors deter the woman from responding to her sexual partner, intercourse may be painful because she is not getting properly aroused by him.

### 2 Decrease in muscular tone

When the level of hormones becomes too low, the muscles of the genitalia and surrounding structures lose their proper tone, and so the vagina may become patulous and a condition of prolapse may result, the uterus dropping, and a cystocele or rectocele may develop. Pessaries and rings can be fitted to support the sagging structures, but in severe cases remedial surgery may be necessary.

## 3 Oestrogen deficiency causing lowered mood and sexual disinterest

Sexual difficulties can develop as a secondary effect of a woman's lowered mood resulting from oestrogen deficiency. This is a controversial issue, but Utian (1978) has put forward this view, and there is, as yet, no definitive evidence on the point. Lowered mood causing sexual unresponsiveness can arise from a number of other factors, including those which are entirely psychological, but there is certainly a case for considering hormone replacement therapy with patients who are somewhat depressed and complaining of sexual disinterest.

## 4 Anorgasmia

When a woman who has previously experienced orgasms either regularly or occasionally becomes anorgasmic in her postmenopausal years, physiological changes may be implicated as well as, or alternatively to, psychogenic factors associated with ageing. Anorgasmia in the female is the neurophysiological equivalent of absent ejaculation in the male, and the organic causes may the same as for the male. Certainly diabetes may produce it, for diabetic neuropathy of the sensory nerves of the clitoris and surrounding structures may inhibit orgasm (Kaplan, 1979).

As in the male, the various drugs that are increasingly prescribed to patients in their later years may have the effect of lowering the sexual response of women and inhibiting orgasm. According to Friedman (1988) 'Anticholinergic drugs, alpha adrenergic receptor blockers, ganglion-blocking drugs and one of the thoxanthines (thioridazine) delay orgasm. Some women complain of anorgasmia on thiazide diuretics'. Dr Whitehead's list of drugs given in Chapter 1 (Table 1.4) was given principally with regard to avoiding the iatrogenic inhibition of penile erection, but they also bear a relationship to the comparable phenomena in the female, as does the whole discussion in the seminar relating to it (Barber *et al.*, 1989a). Amoxapine, an antidepressant drug sometimes prescribed for the elderly, was specifically mentioned by Dr Whitehead in that seminar as inhibiting orgasm in women.

## 5 Hysterectomy and oophorectomy

The risk of needing either or both of these two operations increases with age, and can be compared with risk of prostatectomy in the ageing man. The effects of hysterectomy, as with mastectomy, are mainly psychological. Oophorectomy removes a source of androgens and oestrogens that is still significant, even in the postmenopausal woman, and can be expected to intensify the changes noted above, although in some postmenopausal women the effect is minimal (Weideger, 1977).

## ADVICE AND THERAPY FOR POST-MENOPAUSAL WOMEN

### The role of different professionals

As with men, the main and essential aspect of advice and therapy from all kinds of health-care professionals concerns giving the individual adequate instruction in the facts of sexuality in later life. This chapter has concentrated on outlining the physiological details of the normal processes of ageing, and the abnormalities that may develop and cause problems, because unless people understand what is happening to their own bodies they may be incapable of adjusting emotionally and physically.

Although women who wish for advice and therapy often turn to their GPs, physicians are not always the primary source of care for those in need of help and counselling about their emotional and sexual problems. Vetter *et al.* (1986) describe a scheme in which a health visitor attached to a general practice visited 296 patients aged over 70 years, the scheme extending over two years. They discovered that a surprisingly large number of emotional and physical problems were revealed in patients who had not consulted their doctors. A survey of how often people over the age of 65 visited their doctors was carried out by Luker (1988) on a stratified random sample of 1400 men and women living in Trafford, Manchester. About half of them had not visited their GP with any problem in the last three months before interview, but in the month preceding, 9.6% of their homes had been visited by district nurses and .06% by health visitors. That many old people do not consult their GPs very often can, to some extent, be regarded as a favourable sign of continuing good health, but it may also indicate that for some older people it is a sign of resignation and acceptance of problems that they will talk about to a visiting nurse, but not take to a doctor. The sexual problems of older women are in a special category, as many of them, particularly those of lower socio-economic background, were reared in a climate of acceptance that in the postmenopausal years a woman should not expect to have a rewarding sex-life.

All non-medical health-care professionals need to be aware of the sort of medical conditions that may arise with ageing in order that they should know when to advise people to see their doctors. However, many of the problems that present can be dealt with effectively by simpler counselling, moral support and informing people where to go for help at specialized agencies, a list of which is given in Appendix B. Advice on reading matter is also helpful; more educated people can be advised to read the books by Masters and Johnson (1966; 1970) to give them a basic grasp of the nature of the sexual response and its problems, but there are simple books addressed to the lay public and more suitable for less sophisticated people such as those listed in Appendix A. Doctors' surgeries will thus be spared the attendance of many people whose problems are social and psychological rather than medical.

Sex therapy as such is a matter for specialists and generally involves behaviour therapy and psychotherapy concerned with sexual disorders that have a psychogenic component that is primary, or is secondary to a physiological condition. Sex therapy in the UK (Cole and Dryden, 1988a; Hawton, 1985) is largely geared to the problems of the young and middle-aged, and therapists have tended to apply methods of treatment to older people that are not always appropriate because of the greater degree of physiological involvement in the later years.

## At the doctor's surgery

Doctors should be ready to take an adequate sexual history from their women patients. Asking questions about their patients' sex life should be tactfully geared to general questions about their health as a matter of course, whatever the complaint is that has brought the older woman to the surgery. Sarrel gives the following advice:

> Clarifying the problem not only helps in thinking about what sort of help is indicated, it is a way of telling a woman that her concerns about sex are appropriate, and that the health care provider regards sexual concerns as important, that sex is not a taboo subject to talk about and, by including informed questions, demonstrates some capacity to be helpful (Sarrell, 1988, p. 72).

Taking the sexual history will naturally include questions about vaginal dryness among other post-menopausal symptoms, painful intercourse and lack of normal desire, and comparison of the patient's present sexual feelings with those she had in her pre-menopausal years. The doctor may initiate discussion about the sex life of the spouse, and inquire whether he is having any difficulties. Many of women's problems arise, of course, through their partner's sexual dysfunction, pyschologically or physiologically, and a woman may be urged to get her man to come to the doctor's surgery for advice and possible treatment. Masters and Johnson always tried to treat sexual dysfunction by interviewing couples rather than individuals, but this may not always be appropriate, as some women and men prefer to admit to a doctor or other health-care professional in confidence things that they do not want to admit to their spouse.

In dealing with older women, doctors will be seeing many more who are widowed or divorced, as well as those who have always been single, and some of them may be very reluctant to admit that they have a sex-life, either actually or potentially. By taking it for granted that most women, whatever their marital status, will have sexual urges and a perfect right to enjoy a satisfying sex life, 'permission' will be given to the patient to admit to, and discuss, that side of her life. Although a percentage of women do not, and perhaps never have, masturbated, it is better to ask 'If you masturbate, do you . . . ?' rather than prefacing an inquiry with 'Do you masturbate?', as such a question might imply that the doctor thinks that it is an abnormal practice fraught with danger, as used to be believed. Some women will, of course, be perfectly happy to lead a single, sex-less life, but such evidence that we have indicates that they are a small minority. The knowledge that women after the menopause do not cease to be feminine, sexually attractive and capable, will be a great moral boost to some, even if circumstances dictate that they have no regular or occasional partner.

Physical examination may reveal conditions that need further investigation before an adequate diagnosis can be made and treatment initiated. The main diagnostic decision to be made is whether any difficulties complained of are due to purely psychological and social factors, including the incapacity of the spouse, or whether there is a physiological abnormality to be treated. The levels of serum FHS and ostradiol can be measured, and such measures, taken in conjunction with an observation of genital atrophy and complaints of vaginal drynes, must be taken into account when considering whether to advise hormone replacement therapy.

The GP will not have time for other than brief sexual counselling, but doctors are generally the agency for referring patients in need to other professionals, including specialists in sex therapy, both medical and non-medical.

## Hormonal replacement therapy

Apart from providing reliable information about the normal changes to be expected with ageing, and giving encouragement to continue leading a fulfilling sex-life, the professional health-care provider, when confronted with the problems of ageing men, is largely concerned with problems of failing penile efficiency. The problems of ageing women are quite different with regard to physiology. They revolve round the relatively sudden change in the hormonal system with the menopause, and the question of hormonal replacement therapy has to be considered.

This question has a curious history. Considerable controversy was caused by the pulication of *Feminine Forever*, a book by Wilson (1966), written in over-enthusiastic terms and seemingly promising a golden future for postmenopausal women by means of oestrogen therapy, even though at that time the effects of exogenous oestrogen had not been fully researched. The controversy that ensued can be viewed with hindsight in the light of a very old controversy within medical science: how far is it desirable to use 'artificial' means to prevent the pains and tribulations to which the human body is subject through 'natural' processes? This controversy flourished in the early days of attempts to introduce anaesthesia in surgery, some opponents of the practice claiming that surgical patients recovered quicker if they suffered the 'natural' penalty of pain. A little later it was argued that while anaesthesia might be permissible for surgery, it was certainly not for women in childbed, for giving birth was a natural female function and they must expect to suffer pain. The arguments against providing postmenopausal women with hormonal replacement were considerably more sophisticated and reasonable, but they had overtones of this age-old controversy in medicine. How far should medical science interfere with 'nature'?

The arguments against Wilson's brash optimism were twofold: first, the exogenous hormone might produce cancer in those tissues that have oestrogen receptors, notably the breast and the endometrium of the uterus; second, it was treating women in the postmenopausal years – perhaps a third of a their lives – as though they were suffering from a deficiency disease, and this was considered to be an unwarranted use of medical science.

With regard to the risk of cancer, it was already known that large doses of oestrogen given to mice gave rise to cancers in the reproductive system, but it was not for some years that carefully controlled scientific studies published in *The New England Journal of Medicine* (Zeil and Finkle, 1975; Smith *et al.*, 1975) showed that there was a link between medically prescribed oestrogen and endometrial cancer. The evidence concerning the association between exogenous oestrogen and breast cancer was less clear. A study by Hoover *et al.* (1976) appeared to establish such a link, and led to further research into this question. Gambrell (1987) reviews such research and finally states that 'Numerous studies on oestrogen replacement therapy have failed to incriminate the use of exogenous oestrogen as a cause of breast cancer in postmenopausal women' (p. 123).

Later research on the risk of oestrogen replacement therapy causing endometrial cancer showed that it could be reduced by the cyclic addition of progesterone (Jensen *et al.*, 1987). All medical treatment involves certain risks for some individuals, and policy must be determined by balancing the iatrogenic risks against the naturally occurring risks, and an excellent discussion of this question with respect to hormone replacement herapy is given by Utian (1988). He sums up the present position thus:

> It is still not practical to recommend long-term hormonal-therapy for all women after the menopause. Rather, alterations in lifestyle, including nutritional advice, physical therapy and exercise guidance, and a planned osteoporosis screening programme are of prime importance.
>
> These women requesting long-term HRT on an individual basis, provided they are well informed, should not be refused such therapy. (Utian, 1988, pp. 268–269).

The physician will, of course, be aware of the contraindications in individual cases, such as a history of diabetes, high blood pressure, coronary thrombosis, cancer of breast, uterus or ovaries, obesity, and never having been pregnant.

If we admit that with modern treatments, hormonal replacement therapy is safe if carefully administered and medically monitored, there is still the argument that it may be treating the post-menopausal state as though it were a deficiency disease rather than recognizing it as a natural phase in a woman's life. But the question is, how 'natural' is it? Until modern techniques of preventive and remedial medicine evolved, relatively few women lived to enjoy a post-menopausal span of life, for the expectation of life was around that of the menopause. We have created a period of life during which the emotional, physical and social quality of living is seriously handicapped for many women, and it would seem logical that if medical science has created a human problem for many individuals by interfering with 'natural' death-dealing factors, science should provide the remedy, just as it does for those unlucky enough to become diabetic.

There are some specialists in hormone replacement therapy who regard the medical profession as a whole as being too reluctant to take action when it is appropriate. Thus Greenblatt (1988) writes as follows:

> Too many fear that oestrogens are responsible for mammary and uterine cancers and ignore the benefits which far outweigh the risks. Actually the incidence of endometrial cancers has

been reduced to less than the natural incidence of the disease whenever a sequential oestrogen-progestogen regimen has been utilized. By shunning hormone replacement, the complications of such treatment are avoided and the physician detaches himself from any blame should a gynaecic neoplasm appear. Brave new world! Surely, 'do no harm' and 'benign neglect' are not mutually exclusive. *Nolle nocere* is not a mandate not to attempt to do good. (Greenblatt, 1988, viii).

### The interaction between emotional and physiological factors

The process of physiological sexual arousal depends upon emotional factors, and there is presumably a feed-back loop in the neurological system whereby the arousal builds up by such interaction. However, the extent to which the long-term physiological status of a woman's sexual system is dependent on her emotional life is not clear. There is also a lack of precise knowledge about the cause–effect relationship between continued sexual activity and the degree of atrophy, both physiological and anatomical, that may occur in the postmenopausal years. A number of research studies have validated the common saying that 'if you don't use it you lose it' with respect to sexuality, but there is anecdotal evidence of people in later life who, after years of sexual abstinence, fall in love and form very satisfactory sexual relationships. Leiblum *et al.* (1983) have studied the question of the extent to which continued sexual activity can prevent the atrophy of women's genital organs in the post-menopausal years, but there are many emotional and social variables concerned in the continuation of such activity.

One of the disabilities that older women suffer is the shortage of men in their own age-group. Statistics of the great numerical disparity between the sexes is given in Chapter 6, but here we may simply note the fact the this poses a great problem for health-care professionals who counsel older people. It is all very well to suggest to a woman that she might possibly be healthier and happier if she had an active sex life, but what do we advise when she asks 'But where are the men?'

Here the therapist must avoid being put in the position of seeming to be proselytizing, for some people are perfectly healthy and well adjusted who have no sex life at all, and some have social, religious and other objections to some of the alternatives that might be put forward. To consider possible alternatives we may turn to the suggestions advanced by Brecher (1984) in considering the results of his study of 4,246 men and women aged 50–93 years, bearing in mind that it was a biased survey because it was self-selected.

*Solving the dearth-of-men problem*
Despite the shortage of unmarried men, 160 of our unmarried women report an ongoing sexual relationship, and 48 report one or more casual partners last year. Where do they find their sexual partners?

In the sections that follow, we shall discuss four possible solutions in order of their frequency:

First, 40 percent (60) of our unmarried women with ongoing sexual partners have taken a *married* man as a lover.

Next, a substantial but smaller number are making do with a male lover much older than they are.

Third, a surprising number have a much younger male lover.

Finally, there is a solution that is often discussed nowadays but is extremely rare in our sample. With so devastating a shortage of unattached older men, it is asked, why shouldn't older women team up with one another? (Brecher 1984, pp. 176–177).

In the text that follows, it is made clear that by 'teaming up' a sexual lesbian association is meant. In the present climate of opinion, health-care professionals must take a non-judgemental position with regard to the adultery that is involved in the first alternative. With regard to the fourth alternative, the feminist movement have already made lesbianism an acceptable and respected way of life. How far it is advisable to discuss all or any of these alternatives with a woman who is living a celibate life but who hints that she would welcome sexual fulfilment, must depend on the professional acumen of the health-care worker.

It should be realized that however tactfully the question of beginning a sex life is raised with a widowed, divorced, or single woman there may be an immediate rejection of the idea. But such rejection must not be taken as permanent. Unforseen circumstances, such as the meeting of an acceptable lover, may entirely alter a woman's attitude to the situation, and here the non-judgemental attitude of the professional adviser may have a critical effect on the decision a woman makes. She will remember that her social worker, doctor or other adviser did not view such an eventuality as being outside the range of possibilities, or in any way ridiculous whatever her age, and she may therefore embrace a new opportunity for happiness and fulfilment.

Doctors should realize that their medical ministrations may produce an unexpected change in the emotional orientation of a woman with regard to sex. If hormone replacement therapy is initiated in the treatment of some such condition as osteoporosis, it may be that sexual desire will be stimulated in a woman, married or single, who is having no sex life, as sexual fantasies and needs are sometimes re-awakened by the change in the system following hormone replacement therapy (Dow *et al.*, 1983; Sherwin and Gelfand, 1985). Where a woman has been living asexually but contentedly with an impotent husband who is also without desire, a new factor that is potentially disruptive will be introduced into the marriage. What is done in such a situation must depend on the mature judgement of the doctor.

## REFERENCES

Barber, H.R.K., Bulter, R.N., Lewis M., Long, J. and Whitehead, E.D. (1989a) Sexual problems in the elderly. I The use and abuse of medications, *Geriatrics*, 44, 61–71.

Brecher, E.M. (1984), *Love, Sex, and Aging: A Consumer Union Report*, Little, Brown & Co, Boston.

Catania, J.A. and White, C.B. (1982), Sexuality in an ageing sample: cognitive determinants of masturbation, *Arch. Sex. Behav.* 11, 237–245.

Cole, M. and Dryden, W. (1988a) *Sex Therapy in Britain* Open University Press, Milton Keynes.

Cole, M. and Dryden, W. (1988b), Sexual dysfunction: an introduction, in Cole, M. and Dryden, W. (eds) *Sex Therapy in Britain*, pp. 3–11, Open University Press, Milton Keynes.

Cooper, G.F. (1988) The psychological methods of sex therapy, in Cole, M. and Dryden, W. (eds) *Sex Therapy in Britain*, Open University Press, Milton Keynes.

Croft, L.H. (1982) *Sexuality in the Later Years*, John Wright, Boston.

Dalton, K. (1978) *Once a Month*, Fontana, London.

Dow, M., Hart, D. and Forrest, C. (1983) Hormonal treatment of sexual unresponsiveness in postmenopausal women: a comparative study, *Br. J. Obstet. Gynecol.*, 90, 361–366.

Friedman, D. (1988) Assessing the basis of sexual dysfunction: diagnostic procedures, in Cole, M. and Dryden, W. (eds) *Sex Therapy in Britain*, pp. 105–124, Open University Press, Milton Keynes.

Gambrell, R.D. (1987) Hormone replacement therapy and breast cancer, *Maturitas*, 9, 123–133.

Greenblatt, R.B. (1988) Foreword, in Studd, J.W.W. and Whitehead, M.I. (eds.) *The Menopause*, pps vii–viii. Blackwell Publications, Oxford.

Hawton, K. (1985) *Sex Therapy: A Practical Guide*. Oxford University Press, Oxford.

Hegeler, S. and Mortensen, M.M. (1978) Sexual behavior in elderly Danish males. In Gemme, R. and Wheeler, C.C. (eds) *Progress in Sexology: Selected Papers from the proceedings of the 1976 International Congress of Sexology*, Plenum Press, New York.

Hoover, R., Gray, L.A., Cole, P. and McMahon, B. (1976) Menopausal estrogen and breast cancer, *New Eng. J. Med*, 295, 401–405.

Jaszmann, L. (1973), Epidemiology of the climacteric and post-climacteric complaints, in Van Keep, P.A. and Lauritzen, C. (eds) *Ageing and Oestrogens*, pp. 22–25. Klarger, Basel.

Jensen, P.B., Jensen, J., Riis, B.J., Rodbro, P., Strom, V. and Christiansen, C. (1987) Climacteric symptoms after oral and percutaneous replacement therapy, *Maturitas*, 9, 207–215.

Kaplan, H.S. (1979) *Disorders of Sexual Desire*, Baillière Tindall, London.

Kaufert, P.A., Gilbert, P. and Tate, R. (1987) Defining menopausal status: the impact of longitudinal data, *Maturitas*, 9, 217–226.

Kinsey, A.C., Pomeroy, W.B., Martin, C.E. and Gebhard, P.H. (1953) *Sexual Behavior in the Human Female*, W.B. Saunders, Philadelphia.

Leiblum, S.R., Bachmann, G.A. Kemmann, E. Colburn, D. and Schwartzman, L. (1983) Vaginal atrophy in post-menopausal women, *J.Am. Med. Ass.* 249, 2195–2198.

Levin. R.J. (1981) The female orgasm – a current research, *J. Psychosom. Res.*, 25, 119–133.

Luker, K. (1988) The nurse's role in health promotion and preventive health care of the elderly, in Wells, N. and Freer, C. (eds.) *The Ageing Population: Burden or Challenge?* pp. 155–161, The Macmillan Press, Basingstoke.

Masters, W.H. and Johnson, V.E. (1966), *Human Sexual Response*. Little, Brown & Co, Boston.

Masters, W.H. and Johnson, V.E. (1970) *Human Sexual Inadequacy*, J. & A. Churchill, London.

Morris, N.M and Udry, J.R. (1975) *An Experimental Search for Pheromonal Influences on Human Sexual Behavior*, Eastern Conference on Reproductive Behavior, Nags Head N.C.

Neugarten, B.L., Wood, V. and Kraines, R. (1968) Women's attitudes toward the menopause, in Neugarten, B. (ed.) *Middle Age and Aging*, University of Chicago Press, Chicago.

Newman, G. and Nichols, C.B. (1960) Sexual activities and attitudes in older persons, *J.Am. Med. Ass.* 173, 33–35.

Pfeiffer, E., Verwoerdt, A. and Davis, G.C. (1972) Sexual behavior in middle life, *Am. J. Psychiat.* 128, 1262–1267.

Riley, A.J. (1988) The endocrinology of sexual function and dysfunction, in Cole, M. and Dryden, W. (eds) *Sex Therapy in Britain*, pp. 69–90. Open University Press, Milton Keynes.

Sarrel, P.M. (1988) Sexuality, in Studd, J.W.W. and Whitehead, M.I. (eds) *The Menopause*, pp. 65–75, Blackwell Scientific Publications, Oxford.

Sherwin, B.B. and Gelfand, M.M. (1985) Differential symptom response to parenteral estrogen and/or androgen administration in the surgical menopause, *Am. J. Obstet. Gynecol.* 151, 153–160.

Smith, D.C., Prentice, R., Thompson, D.J. and Herrman, W.L. (1975) Association of exogenous estrogen and endometrial carcinoma, *New Eng. J. Med.* 293, 1164–1167.

Starr, B.D. and Weiner, M.B. (1981) *The Starr-Weiner Report on Sex and Sexuality in the Mature Years*, McGraw Hill, New York.

Utian, W.H. (1988) Analysis of hormone replacement therapy, in Studd, J.W.W. and Whitehead, M.I. (eds) *The Menopause*, pp. 262–270, Blackwell Scientific Publications, Oxford.

Van Keep, P.A. and Kellerhals, J.M. (1974) The impact of sociocultural factors on symptom formation, *Psychother. Psychosom.*, 23, 251–263.

Verwoerdt, A., Pfeiffer, E. and Wang, H.S. (1969) Patterns of sexual activity and interest, *Geriatrics*, 24, 137–154.

Vetter, N.J., Jones, D.A. and Victor, C.R. (1986) A health visitor affects the problems others do not reach, *The Lancet*, 2, 30–32.

Waslow, M. and Loeb, M. (1975) Sexuality in nursing homes, *J.Am. Geriat. Soc.* 27, 73–79.

Weidiger, P. (1977) *Female Cycles*, The Women's Press, London.

White, C.B. (1982) Sexual interest, attitude, knowledge and sexual history in relation to sexual behavior in the institutionalized aged, *Arch. Sex. Behav.* 11, 11–21.

Wilson, G.D. (1988) The psychobiological basis of sexual dysfunction, in Cole M. and Dryden, W. (eds) *Sex Therapy in Britain*. pp 49–68. Open University Press, Milton Keynes.

Wilson, R.A. (1966) *Feminine Forever*, Evans, New York.

Winn, R.L. and Newton, N. (1982) Sexuality in aging: a study of 106 cultures, *Archiv. Sex. Behav.* 11, 283–298.

Ziel, H.K. and Finkle, W.D. (1975) Increased risk of endometrial carcinoma among users of conjugated estrogens, *New Eng. J. Med.* 293, 1167–1170.

# 3

# Psychosocial factors affecting the emotional lives of older people

When we refer to the emotional lives of people, we mean their whole view of themselves, how they relate to other people and the world about them. Are they generally happy or sad – self-confident or timid – out-going or reserved – affectionate or cold? As will be discussed later, many of the stereotypes of ageing depict it as a period of growing disenchantment with living, and life becoming a burden, as expressed so eloquently in the *Book of Ecclesiastes*:

> Remember now thy Creator in the days of thy youth, while the evil days come not, nor the years draw nigh, when thou shalt say, I have no pleasure in them.

The case is presented in this chapter that the stereotype of the elderly that is generally held in this, or any other society, is of very great importance for the happiness and physical welfare of older people. If society has a generally negative stereotype of elderly people, then as we all grow older we shall expect to become like that one day, and it may become a self-fulfilling prophecy. According to Comfort (1990) while 25% of the disabilities of elderly people are biogenic and depend on medical science for their alleviation or cure, 75% are sociogenic, and their remedy depends on changed attitudes on the part of society, and of the people themselves.

For reasons that will be discussed later in this book, there has been a relatively sudden surge in the size of the population in the older decades of life, and we are confronted with problems that have never been encountered before in the history of humanity. All health-care workers, whatever their specialism, are having to re-think many of their traditional practices and assumptions in response to the new challenges, and in the light of new research findings. This chapter concentrates on examining the different sources of the stereotypes we hold about older people, and the ideas we may have adopted, perhaps unthinkingly, which can condition and even hamper us in our approach to the problems we have to address in our professional work.

## The unrepresentative minorities that health-care professionals see

Here it is appropriate to make the point that health-care professionals may get a biased and pessimistic view of older people, and indeed, of society in general, because they are constantly concerned with the various sorts of casualties of society, the unhealthy, the maladjusted and the atypical. Freer (1988) points out some of the reasons why both professionals and the lay public are likely to form an all too pessimistic view of the prevalence of problems among older people. It is for this reason we shall present throughout this book the results of a wide range of research among normal people, those who seldom or never come to the attention of health-care professionals. This is very necessary when we are dealing with the older section of the population, for otherwise we may make the mistake of equating ageing with disability, and promote the unfortunate stereotype that is so damaging to older people. We must keep in mind that despite all the factors, both biogenic and sociogenic, that make life difficult in later life, most older people in our society are pretty healthy, and, married or single, living quite rewarding lives. The study by Luker and Perkins (1987) in Manchester showed that over 90 per cent of elderly people questioned rated their health as being from fair to good. If we are well-informed about the lives of the normal majority, we are in a better position to help the minority who are in need of care.

### THE MEDICAL STEREOTYPE OF THE ELDERLY

Freer expresses the medical stereotype of older people that is held all too frequently when he writes,

It is likely that when asked to think of an old person, most of us, whether lay or professional, are likely to picture a frail, bent person, slow to move and think and short of memory.

More specific medical stereoypes such as incontinence, dementia and deafness are also likely to spring to mind. As with many commonly held beliefs there is some basis for this one. The prevalence of disease and dependency problems is higher in the over-65-year-old age group, and the frequency of reported health problems increases with advancing years. (Freer, 1988, p. 3).

However, although the frequency of such problems is higher in the later years of life, it is easy to get a biased view of the situation that does not accord with the facts. It is possible that the professional stereotype in this matter is rather more gloomy than the lay stereotype, for if one is chiefly concerned with the section of the elderly population who are ill-housed, impoverished, unhealthy, and in need of professional help, it is natural to equate age with deterioration. But if most of the elderly one comes across are going on binges to Blackpool, coach trips to the Costa Brava, or attending the classes and activities of The University of the Third Age, a very different image is conveyed. Here there is a certain confusion among professional people between *geriatrics* and *gerontology*. Some writers have even referred to 'geriatric sex' when they mean lovemaking between older people! Geriatrics have taught us much about the illnesses and disabilities that are more common in the later years of life, but research in social gerontology, a much younger discipline, has thrown some much-needed light on the realities of ageing for the population in general.

In a study of general practice, Wilkin and Williams (1986) found that while patients over 75 years were 6% of their study population, they accounted for only 8% of the consultations. While this comparatively low percentage may represent a certain amount of under-consultation, as studied by Ford and Taylor (1985), it does not support the pessimistic image of the elderly as depicted in the passage quoted above. Research data from the Aldermore Health Centre (cited by Freer, 1988) provides some interesting information about the frequency of consultations of 8,423 people over the whole age range up to 99 years. While up to the age of 64 years there was a mean yearly consultation rate of 2.8% (including surgery and home visits) the increase half-decade by half-decade thereafter was very gradual and had reached only 4.7% by the age of 89 years.

One might expect that, as the number of elderly people in the population is steadily increasing, the demands on doctors' surgeries would be getting more and more, but this does not appear to be the case. Wilson (1982) found that the demands by the elderly section of the population on medical services had not increased over a period of 18 years. In the Aldermoor Health Centre data referred to above, while the average yearly consultation rate was 2.8% for those under 65 years, the rate rose to only 2.9% if 845 older people are added to the computation. Demands will, of course, vary from district to district, but the question arises, as the number of the elderly increases, are they getting more and more healthy, generation by generation, and more independent of health-care professionals? Fries (1980), whose work will be discussed later, proposed that 'the number of very old persons will not increase, that the average period of diminished physical vigour will decrease, that chronic disease will occupy a smaller proportion of the typical lifespan, and that the need for medical care in later life will decrease' (p. 130). If such an aim is feasible, we should do all we can to achieve it, and studying the emotional foundations of healthy living is highly relevant.

**The myth versus the reality**

The question posed above is very complex, and it will be a long time before any clear answers will be forthcoming. It may be that if less freely available medical care is available, more demands will be made on social workers and other non-medical health-care givers, and vice-versa. We have to consider what we mean by 'health'. Surprisingly it has been found that what is more important than objective assessments of fitness, as by social workers' assessments, medical diagnoses, etc., is the individual's own assessment of his or her well-being. In a large research study Mossey and Shapiro (1982) found that the best predictor of longevity was the individual's self-perception of well-being. This study concerned 3,128 non-institutionalized residents of Manitoba, and it indicated that even though people might be suffering from various objectively identifiable disabilities, including low income and indifferent health, it was their *subjective* rating of their fitness that was the important predictor of longevity. Coleman (1983) has also referred to similar evidence from a German study carried out by Thomae that it is the emotional health of older people, their positive perception of themselves, that is of primary importance in maintaining their continued well-being. In fact, a number of research studies have shown that for most elderly people there is no evidence that getting older significantly reduces their happiness and self-perceived health, provided that they have sufficient factors in their lives that maintain their morale. Given an adequately satisfying emotional life, they will adapt to adverse conditions, such as the stiffening of the joints with arthritis, and continue to lead as full lives as before.

Men and women differ in a number of important ways as they age. For instance, it has been found that while the married state is correlated with continued good health and longevity for both sexes, it is more protective for men than for women (Gove, 1973). Thus, as far as men, the weaker vessels, are concerned, they are fortunate in having a greater choice of marital partners in later life because of the numerical imbalance of the sexes! Both sexes need to love and be loved, but men are more dependent on their masculine self-image being maintained.

**The rectangular survival curve**

The stereotype that younger people, both professional and lay, have of ageing includes a false model of deterioration over time. It is supposed that older people's health and general abilities steadily decay until eventually they die, worn out by living. Such a false stereoype, as it exists in America, is extensively criticised in Harris' (1975) book. Superficially such a model can be sustained on the basis of cross-sectional research. Thus if we compare the average fitness of groups of people aged 60–64, 65–69, 70–74 . . . etc. we will get a steadily descending curve, and such a gradient of declining fitness is what many people imagine to be the case in the life of any individual. But this descending curve is an artefact of the group averages, since in any group there will be people 'on their last legs' and about to die. Such cases pull down the arithmetical average for the group, and as we all must die sometime, the higher we go up the age-scale, the more of such cases there will be.

A truer picture is conveyed by longitudinal research, that is, studying the same individuals over time. Such research shows that for most of us a fairly steady plateau of health is maintained for quite a span of years before the eventual demise. This was found, for example, in Maddox's (1981) study of measuring the well-being of people in the later decades of life. It was found that older people functioned at much the same level over quite a long period of time, suffering the usual ups and downs of health that are experienced at all ages, but not deteriorating as is popularly supposed. Obviously the sheer luck of life events determines increases and decreases of well-being: in the Duke University study (Pfeiffer *et al.* 1968) some men actually increased their sexual activity after the age of 70, and Chirikos and Nestel (1985) found that a substantial proportion of individuals who suffered from various disabilities improved their functional status as they grew older.

This brings us to the remarkable paper by Fries (1980) which was mentioned earlier, in which he maintained that the number of very old persons in society will not increase over time, and that the average period of diminished vigour in people's lives will become smaller, and so the need for medical care and other dependency in later life will actually *decrease* as time goes on. This controversial claim will be considered further in the last chapter of this book where we try to project into the 21st century, but for the moment it will suffice to point out one salient feature of Fries' theory. He postulates what he calls a 'rectangular survival curve' that can be contrasted with the popular assumption of a steadily descending curve in later life. One of his less well-founded speculations is that the 'natural' span of our lives is 85 years, so that, with little but adequate social and medical support we should expect to maintain pretty good health and vigour until that age, then suddenly 'drop off our perches'. This is, of course, an over-simplified account of Fries's thesis, but it is worth presenting here, in order to contrast it with a more complex model of human development in the later years which emphasizes that it is mistake to consider 'old people' as a homogenous group. It may be that different individuals are genetically programmed to be long lived or short lived, although environmental factors of disease, accident, nutrition etc. will play a powerful part in longevity. As yet, research is not sufficiently advanced to tell us much about this, but we may, by analogy, refer to the fact that females who have an early menarch tend to have a late menopause, and vice-versa, irrespective of the environmental factors during the years of fertility (Dalton, 1978). The concept of 'elite survivors' has been discussed by some gerontologists, and it has been pointed out that:

> Grouping together cohorts born in different environments as 'the elderly' may be administratively convenient but less than satisfactory for the development of more sensitive policies and appropriate research. The presence of considerable heterogeneity among older populations and the need for this to be recognised in research is thus underlined (Bury, 1988, p. 29).

**Implications for professional workers**

All the above questions need to be considered by professional workers in their interaction with clients and patients. The extent to which the attitude of the professional worker influences the self-image of those in receipt of any sort of care is unknowable, but is probably very important indeed. It should never be assumed that because a person was born in a certain year he or she will 'naturally' suffer from this or that disability, or should not attempt a particular line of action because it is too demanding or inappropriate after a certain age. People should be made aware of the known risk-factors associated with different age-groups, but it is up to them whether or not they are prepared to take such risks. It is apparent that the 'medical stereotype' of ageing is changing, and we should be alive to these changes. Before we consider further how such changes will affect our practice in the future it is necessary to take a more general look at the various sources of how ageing is viewed in the society we live in.

**AGE IDENTIFICATION**

When addressing people over the age of 60 years, professional people should be very careful as to how they refer to their age-status. A surprisingly large number of such people will be slightly offended if they are referred to as 'elderly' or 'old'. The unthinking

**Table 3.1** Reasons given for personal age identification

| Identification as young or middle-aged (N = 148) | Number[a] | Percentage | Identification as elderly or old (N = 172) | Number[a] | Percentage |
|---|---|---|---|---|---|
| Still active and busy | 85 | 59.8 | Particular health problem (e.g., heart attack) | 49 | 28.5 |
| Good physical and/or mental health | 84 | 59.1 | | | |
| Positive mental attitude | 41 | 28.9 | Retirement | 38 | 22.1 |
| Rapport with young people | 20 | 14.1 | Physical slowdown (e.g., tire easily) | 35 | 20.3 |
| Youthful appearance | 12 | 8.4 | Health restrictions | 22 | 12.8 |
| Mix with all ages | 12 | 8.4 | Just age (no other reason) | 20 | 11.6 |
| Can still handle own affairs | 10 | 7.0 | Change in social contacts | 10 | 5.8 |
| Other | 10 | 7.0 | Illness or death of spouse | 10 | 5.8 |
| | | | Other | 26 | 15.1 |

[a] Each respondent could give more than one response.
Table from *The Aging Experience* by Russell A. Ward. Copyright © 1979 by J.B. Lippincott Company. Reprinted by permission of HarperCollins Publishers.

reference to 'An old lady like you . . .' may be displeasing to a woman in her seventies who does not regard herself as 'an old lady'. Some data relevant to this come from a survey by Ward (1979) in which he interviewed 320 men and women in the age cohorts of the 60s, 70s and 80s. They were asked how they would classify themselves with respect to their age-status, and while 172 referred to themselves as 'elderly' or 'old', 148 saw themselves as 'young' or 'middle-aged'. How such a question is posed makes quite a lot of difference, but it was clear that some of them even in the oldest age cohort, did not regard themselves as being 'old'. This study investigated the reasons why people would see themselves as being in one or the other category, and a summary of the reasons are shown in Table 3.1.

It will be seen from Table 3.1 that the principal determinants of older people's perception of their age-status are health and productive activity. Thus sickly men or women in their early 60s, who have retired from work and have no particular occupation, may regard themselves as 'elderly or old', whereas healthy people in their 80s who are still busily occupied, either gainfully or voluntarily, may still see themselves as no more than 'middle-aged', and may indeed have long ago given up bothering about their age.

When they get to a certain age, quite a number of people realize that the whole business of age-status is rather an illusion. All their lives they had expected to be 'old' when they reached a certain date on the calendar, but when they reached it they did not feel any different. They realized that they were still 'young' in their inner being and perception of themselves. Occasionally a man in his 80s may say that when he attends gatherings of retired people, some much younger than himself, he looks around the grey heads and wrinkled faces, and thinks to himself 'Poor old fellows – I'm glad I'm not like them!' Simone de Beauvoir (1972) observed that 'old people are also mirrors for one another, mirrors in which they do not care to see themselves – the marks of old age they behold vex them' (p. 472). The viewer sees the externals, and because of his long conditioning by society's stereotypes of age, he cannot realize that many of these people feel just like he does in their inner selves.

It is important for professional people who come in contact with those who have lived a relatively long time, to keep in mind that their concern is with problems to do with health, housing, finance, family difficulties, etc., and not with age as such. The age of a person is no excuse for being less efficient and energetic in trying to solve problems, than in the case of younger people. It might seem that this hardly needs pointing out, but there is a slight tendency for older people to be treated differently because it is thought that in certain areas of life their needs are less important than those of younger people. Norman (1987) commented on the fact that some 'social workers felt that elderly people, as compared with children, have had their lives and have no future contribution to make to society, so why bother with them?' (p. 10). There is a story of a man aged 103 who went to his doctor complaining that his right knee was rather stiff, and demanding treatment. The doctor saw that he was not seriously incapacitated and, being unable to suggest any useful treatment, took refuge in saying 'Well, that knee is 103 years old, so I don't see you have much to complain of.' The patient replied, 'Well the left knee is also 103 years old and it's all right – so what are you going to do about the right one?'

The fact that a client or patient looks 'old' and is indeed a very senior citizen according to the date of birth, does not mean that he or she is in any way different, intellectually, emotionally or socially, from younger people. Much depends upon the individual. Although we have just discussed how health determines, to some extent, people's perception of themselves with respect to age-status, health is a relative matter. One can be sickly at any age, yet still feel and act with vigour intellectually and emotionally. It was noted in Chapter 1 that in Brecher's (1984) study among people of quite advanced years a remarkably large proportion of both men and women reported being sexually active, and with a high enjoyment of sex – despite being in only fair or poor health, and despite the seven adverse health factors that were reviewed. The fact that some people in the last decades of their life take up totally new careers, develop fresh and absorbing interests, fall in love, and give other signs of that intangible quality of a 'positive mental attitude', as mentioned in Table 3.1, is evidence that the potential for living life to the full need not evaporate with age.

Pablo Casals, the great Spanish musician, said the following when interviewed at the age of ninety-three:

> On my last birthday I was ninety-three years old. That is not young of course. . . . But age is a relative matter. If you

continue to work and to absorb the beauty of the world about you, you find that age does not necessarily mean getting old. At least, not in the ordinary sense. I feel many things more intensely than before, and for me life grows more fascinating. . . .

Work helps prevent one from getting old. I, for one, cannot dream of retiring. Not now or ever. Retire, the word is alien and the idea inconceivable to me. My work is my life. I cannot think of one without the other. To 'retire' means to me to begin to die. The man who works and is never bored is never old. Work and interest in worthwhile things are the best remedy for age. Each day I am reborn. Each day I must begin again (From Kahn, 1970, pp. 15–17).

The great problem before us is how health care professionals can best promote the potential of ageing people for living life to the full until the day of their death.

## DISENGAGEMENT THEORY

Disengagement theory holds that it is desirable and almost inevitable that at a certain age people should distance themselves from participation and concern with the ordinary life of the community, both occupationally, socially and psychologically, and retire to a life that is more private, and more restricted. In India there is a Hindu tradition of elderly people giving up all responsibility and retiring to an ascetic way of life, spending their time in contemplative pursuits and visiting sacred shrines, thus preparing themselves for life in a future world after death. Such a tradition does not embrace the great mass of the very poor in India, for whatever limited capacity may remain to them can be put to some use in poor communities. Merriman (1984) describes how the old are looked after in village life, and old women perform tasks of child-minding doing whatever simple work is within their capability. There is no disengagement there. In mediaeval Europe there was a tradition of more affluent people breaking the marriage tie if they had lived to what was then considered old age, and retiring into monasteries and nunneries for the last years of their life.

Much that was written about the disengagement of older

people in the sociological and developmental literature some time ago (Cumming and Henry, 1961; Cumming, 1963), was based on a self-fulfilling prophesy, to some degree. In our modern, secular society individuals have been compelled to disengage because of the social and economic pressures that were put upon them, yet this is not an entirely modern phenomenon. The fate of Shakespeare's King Lear, who felt that he should desengage in favour of his daughters, should be a warning to us all! Disengagement theory holds that the process of giving up rights and responsibilities at a certain age, and retiring to a metaphorical rocking chair, is universal, and moreover, that it is to the advantage of both society and the individual. It hardly needs pointing out that a neurosurgeon cannot operate as effectively in his 50s as when he was younger, just as a coal-heaver cannot heave coal as efficiently after a certain age, but that does not mean that they should disengage either socially or economically as they age and be content to accept a lower standard of living and a less respected place in society. The extent that they are forced to do so is an indictment of the economic and social organization of our society.

Disengagement theory has come in for a good deal of criticism in more recent years. For instance, Hochschild (1975) criticizes the general theory on the grounds that it ignores the various meanings that disengagement and ageing may have for different individuals. It is not a unitary process, for some people may disengage psychologically but not occupationally. Thus a journalist may continue working at his economically rewarding trade in his later years, long after he has disengaged psychologically and socially from the world of journalism, as other spheres of endeavour may have come to capture and absorb his interests. Dowd (1975) points out that disengagement may be most unwelcome for some people, and simply reflect their diminished power, their unwilling withdrawl from interactive exchanges because social institutions such as occupational retirement have robbed them of the rewards they used to have. Comfort (1990) gives a satirical picture of the negative stereotype of the disengaged 'old person' in contemporary society:

> Let us look at the stereotype of the ideal aged person as past folklore presents it. He or she is white haired, inactive, and

unemployed, making no demands on anyone, least of all the family, docile in putting up with the loneliness, cons of every kind and type of boredom, and able to live on a pittance. He or she, although not demented, which would be a nuisance to other people, is slightly deficient in intellect, and tiresome to talk to, because folklore says that old people are weak in the head, asexual, because old people are incapable of sexual activity, and it is unseemly if they are not. He or she is unemployable, because old age is second childhood and everyone knows that the old make a mess of simple work. Some credit points can be gained by visiting or being nice to a few of these subhuman individuals, but most of them prefer their own company and the company of other aged unfortunates. Their main occupations are religion, grumbling, reminiscing and attending the funerals of friends. If sick, they need not, and should not, be actively treated, and are best stored in institutions where they can be supervised by bossy matrons who keep them clean, silent and out of sight. A few, who are amusing or active, are kept by society as pets. The rest are displaying unpardonable bad manners by continuing to live, and even on occasion of complaining of their treatment, when society has declared them unpeople and their patriotic duty is to lie down and die (Comfort, 1990, pp. 21–22).

Although the above is deliberately exaggerated, it contains many important truths. Earlier, we saw that some people, even at quite an advanced age, are highly reluctant to be regarded as 'elderly or old' because of the negative connotations of such terms. The label of being 'old' is an attribute known as a *master status trait* as defined by Becker: 'Possession of one deviant trait may have a generalized symbolic value, so that people automatically assume that its bearer possesses other undesirable traits allegedly associated with it' (Becker, 1963, p. 33). Thus a man over the age of 60 may be perceived not just as someone who happens to have been born on a certain date, but as an 'old person', and therefore presumed to be a bit slow on the uptake, and to possess the various other attributes listed by Comfort in the quoted passage.

Nowadays we hear a lot about the evils of racism and sexism, and there are laws to prevent discrimination on grounds of race and sex. But there are no laws designed to combat ageism.

## THE PUBLIC STEREOTYPE OF THE ELDERLY

**Literature**

The stereotype of older people as displayed in fiction and other literature is important, because all our lives we are subject through our reading to influences that determine how we perceive different groups. Feminist pressure groups have even gone the length of rewriting fairy stories because, they maintain, the traditional ones give an incorrect picture of femininity. The stereotype of the elderly which is conveyed in literature not only determines how the young grow up regarding older people, but it influences how people view themselves as they grow older. As far as Shakespeare represents contemporary Elizabethan concepts of older people, we may turn to a number of his plays for enlightenment.

In Hamlet we have Polonius the subject of the Prince's satire:

Slanders, sir: for the satirical rogue says here, that old men have grey beards; that their faces are wrinkled; their eyes purging thick amber and plum-tree gum; and that they have a plentiful lack of wit, altogether with most weak hams: all of which, sir, though I most powerfully and potently believe, yet I hold it not honesty to have it thus set down; for you yourself, Sir, shall grow old as I am if, like a crab, you could go backward (*Hamlet*, II.ii).

It should be noted that Polonius is not being mocked because he is a rather foolish individual, but because he belongs to the class of 'old men', which is represented as repulsive and stupid, just as in another play Shylock is mocked because he is a Jew.

Elsewhere in Shakespeare's writing, old age in itself is repeatedly depicted as inseparable from folly. In *Much Ado About Nothing* we have Dogberry saying 'A good old man, sir; he will be talking: as they say, "When the age is in the wit is out": God help us!' (III.v). In *The Passionate Pilgrim* we read:

Crabbed age and youth cannot live together:
Youth is full of pleasance, age is full of care;
Youth like summer morn, age like winter weather. . . .
Age I do abhor thee; youth I do adore thee (12).

Many of Shakespeare's sonnets also repeat the refrain of lamenting ageing, and representing it as one of the great sadnesses of life.

So it has been down the ages in literature. In Chaucer we have 'The Merchant's Tale' in which the 'old knight' January (he was 60!) weds a young woman, May, fails to satisfy her sexually and is then cuckolded by her. Boccaccio has similar stories ridiculing old men who try to act like young ones, and the theme is repeated in Restoration drama. Although one can find occasional references to the satisfactions of old age, as in Browning's lines 'Grow old along with me/For the best is yet to be', the overwhelming message is that old age is a horrible spectre, and we show our fear of it by mocking at it, and those who are perceived as 'old'.

Fisher (1977) notes that in twentieth century literature old age is seldom dealt with, and attributes this to the rising 'cult of youth' in which older people are of very little interest or significance. There are important exceptions; notably the novels of Marcel Proust who has plenty of insightful studies of ageing people. Ernest Hemmingway's *Old Man of the Sea* is also unusual in depicting an old man who is young in heart conquering the encroachments of age, but it has very little counterpart in more recent literature. The later part of life is seen by more modern writers as being characterized by weakness, dependence, and lack of dignity. Older people are seen as having no place in the modern world, and black comedies such as Kingsley Amis's *Ending Up* and *The Old Devils* depict people in whom the follies of their younger years are greatly exaggerated and rendered grotesque as they age, as in Muriel Spark's *Memento Mori*. They repeat, in a lesser form, Swift's terrible picture of the Strulbrugs, the unfortunate people who were immortal, in his *Voyage to Laputa*. This creation of Swift's is perhaps the most vicious satire on old age that has ever been written, for not only were the Strulbrugs terribly diseased in body, but were psychologically warped to a degree that no one could show anything but dislike of them, and they were cut off from all reasonable communication with the contemporary world in which they lived. Simone de Beauvoir (1972) suggests that this was partly a bitter self-portrait of Swift in his old age.

The message appears to be that we should not aspire to live beyond middle-age or we shall only make fools of ourselves, and be unable to relate to the modern world. This is a question that must have occurred to most professional people who deal with the elderly, and which is one of the serious issues that the present book attempts to deal with.

De Beauvoir herself, in her book *La Vieillesse*, gives a very negative picture of old age. The book is supposed to be an angry attack on society that mistreats its older citizens, and indeed she says:

> Are the old really human beings? Judging by the way our society treats them, the question is open to doubt. . . . In order to soothe its conscience, our society's ideologists have invented a certain number of myths – myths that contradict one another, by the way – which induce those in the prime of life to see the aged not as fellow men but as another kind of being altogether. The Aged Man is the Venerable Sage who planes high above this mundane sphere. He is an old fool wandering in his dotage. He may be placed above our kind or below it; but in either event he is banished from it. Excluded. But what is thought an even better policy than dressing up the facts is that of taking no notice of them whatsoever – old age is a shameful secret, a forbidden subject. (De Beauvoir 1972).

But De Beauvoir gets carried away by her subject, partly perhaps by her own unhappy personal experience, and by drawing on instances from real life and from fiction, presents a very gloomy picture of old age and old people in her chapter titled 'Old age and everyday life', and elsewhere in the book. In so far as her book has been influential, it has certainly not enhanced the image of old age and old people. Society is castigated for its ill-treatment of its older citizens, but what old horrors most of them are shown to be in De Beauvoir's gallery of old people!

Perhaps there are encouraging signs of a growing recognition of the validity of the aspirations of the old in some literature. Loughman (1983) acknowledges that 'In literature, as well as society, the old who defy the ascetic standard by persevering in acting "young" sexually are treated with scorn.' She gives various examples from Boccaccio, Chaucer, and Congreve, but then goes on to observe that 'Contemporary writers, however, are challenging the old myths and are undermining the stereotypes of the aged.' She gives examples from short stories of four writers, all concerning older men and all with a sexual theme. It may be that this will be a growing theme in the serious literature of the future, and stand in contrast to the pessimism of such writers as Kingsley Amis and Muriel Spark.

## Magazines, popular fiction and advertisements

In Martel's (1968) study of American magazine fiction from 1890–1955, he concluded that there has been a shift from regarding mature middle age as being the prime of life in the late Victorian era, to an idealization of young adulthood. Indeed, in later fiction older characters are seldom mentioned. Studies of the characterization of older people in fiction for adolescents (Peterson and Karnes, 1976), and for children (Selzer and Atchley, 1971), tend to show older people in merely passive roles, divorced from the real concerns of life. In recent years, feminist writers have raged against the depiction of girls and women in a too passively feminine role in fiction, but as yet there has been no movement to alter the ageist trend in literature, and to show older people as other than ciphers. Christine Victor comments:

> Various studies have demonstrated the exclusion of older people from works of fiction; especially those designed for children. Where older characters appear in literature they fulfil a supporting role rather than constituting the central theme of the work. Few literary treatments of the aged tackle the problems of ageing. Rather, old characters are depicted as leading an insulated lifestyle, affecting few people and being affected by few in return. However, there is some evidence that this is changing with the publication of novels dealing with later life, especially as it is experienced by old women (Victor, 1987, pp. 97–98).

It may be argued that children and young people are primarily concerned with the events of youth, and are simply not interested in the concerns of 'the old' (those over 40?) but if we turn to the writers of the last and previous centuries the action certainly contained a good number of older people, whether or not their characters are dealt with sympathetically, and their concerns are as vividly and dramatically represented as those of the younger characters.

While older people, depicted as meaningful characters, tend to be conspicuously absent from many kinds of modern fiction, the subject of ageing tends to have a high prominence in one sort of popular publications – women's magazines. Itzen (1984) reports how she carried out a content analysis of the magazine *Woman* over a six-month period, and found that there was only one issue that did not have a feature article concerned with ageing as it affects women, and most issues had at least two, many having up to four. There were also letters in almost every issue about ageing and attitudes to ageing, plus advice in the 'agony column'. It seems that the coming period of post-menopausal life, with its alleged horrors for the female sex, is being brandished before women as a bogy. It is not questioned that the prospect is pretty horrible; what preoccupies the magazine writers is how to postpone it. It is not difficult to trace the connection between the feature articles and the advertisements. Itzin quotes an advertisement for a skin cream:

Nobody minds if your husband looks his age. Men are lucky. They needn't look young to be still attractive. They often get better looking over the years. Unfortunately the same can't be said for us women. From the first moment a tiny line appears, we need to take extra care of our skins with the special moisturizing treatment. . . . (Itzin, 1984, p. 172).

She describes how the advertisement was illustrated with a man who was wrinkled but handsome, with a wrinkled woman of about the same age beside him, looking alarmed. Her alarm was apparently due to the fact that he was shown smiling and talking to another woman who was unwrinkled! Obviously, it is in the commercial interest of those who sell creams alleged to prevent the natural development of wrinkles, to boost the prevailing paranoia among women about what are perceived to be the ravages of age. It is never asked 'If a man's wrinkled face can be attractive, why cannot a woman's?'

Here we may usefully compare the commercialization of ageism (combined with sexism) with the similarly lucrative exploitation of racism that used to be prevalent in the USA. People of negro ancestry used to be urged to spend money on treatments designed to straighten out their naturally crinkly hair, and to lighten the shade of their skins. This profitable business has now died out owing to the success of the anti-racialist movement, as it is no longer considered unattractive or shameful to have crinkly hair and a dark skin. In fact, some young people of a purely European type are now affecting Afro hairstyles, and crinkling their hair artificially. If we can combat ageism as effectively, perhaps we can look forward to a time when women will line in artificial wrinkles in order to enhance their perceived attractiveness! We should remember the lines in John Donne's poem:

No spring nor summer hath such grace,
As I have seen in one autumnal face.

If magazines for the young and middle-aged pay no attention to the existence of an older age group, what of the commercial interests who can profit from the spending power of this group that is becoming ever more numerous? In 1972 a new magazine was founded, *Retirement Choice*, and in the second issue the President of the Pre-retirement Association, Lord Raglan, wrote protesting that society 'arbitrarily imposes the rules of retirement, and, therefore, society should play its full part in providing pre-retirement education to help people adjust to a new way of life, at what after all is a time of life when change is proverbially difficult.' This heralded an attempt to get people to adopt a new attitude to retirement, and in particular, their habits of spending on consumer goods and services. Women were urged to abandon the old styles of dress that used to be bought by the grandmother generation, and to spend more money on clothes. They were told that 'Now when your husband is going to be at home most of the time, is the moment to make him sit up and take notice of your elegant new image.' (*Retirement Choice*, November 1972, pp. 18–19). This was one of the signs of the growing attempt to change the conservative image and habits of retired people who had previously been all too ready to save their money for the estates that their children would inherit.

This magazine was originally available only to members of the Pre-Retirement Association, but in 1973 it became available to the general public on all bookstalls. It was realized what an enormous potential market there was among people over the age of retirement and the image of the magazine changed. It had glossy covers and went in for publicizing the personalities and faces of older celebrities in show-business, politics and positions of power. The endeavour was to capture a reading public who

69

were about to retire, and then to nurse such readership for the years to come, and so the name was changed to *Pre-Retirement Choice*. Later the title changed again to *Choice* the name which it bears today, and it is now a substantial magazine of nearly 100 pages, advertizing and plugging a new life-style of a freely spending, self-confident class of the 'new old'. The advertisements concentrate on such goods, services, and activities as clothes, foreign travel, gardening, fishing, care of health and looks, and insurance policies. The magazine gives advice on the law, the making of wills, the management of finances and property. The magazine has not yet publicized the new commercial clinics for the treatment of male impotence that have been springing up quite recently and advertising in some newspapers, but no doubt they are being considered.

Two years after this magazine was launched a reader wrote in saying that he had yet to read a letter or article from such people as an agricultural labourer, builder's labourer, factory hand, 'or one of the very large class who on retirement have for income the state pension'. He added, 'My finance will not permit me to indulge in some of the hobbies enjoyed by some of your correspondents.' Another reader wrote in similar vein, saying that 'My guess is that your readers are chiefly those who are getting or will get two pensions.' Two commentators on this magazine write:

> In spite of laudable intentions, the magazine has depended for its survival on fostering specific elements of consumer culture: the cultivation of youthfulness and an energetic outlook, fitness, beauty, self-expression, hedonism, fashion and style. . . . all of which are closely connected with a disposable income; in other words an active role in a market economy. In working towards the dissociation of retirement from late ageing and in effect extending the plateau of active middle age . . . the magazine has had no choice but to ally itself with consumer industries. In a society characterized by socioecomomic changes which do not reward the inactive and the obsolete, one unintended consequence has been the creation of two nations in middle and old age. (Featherstone and Hepworth, 1984, p. 223).

The above is perfectly true. When the Welfare State was launched in the 1940s Richard Titmuss (1959) predicted that

Disraeli's 'Two Nations', would, in the future, come to be a reality for those over the age of retirement, whatever happened to the working population. Magazines such as *Choice* are a powerful force in changing the image of the elderly in contemporary society, but the people with whom professional workers have to deal in providing health care will be mainly those who are less affluent, and have been so all their lives, and therefore have not been greatly affected by this changing image. What will happen in the future remains to be seen, but old attitudes die hard.

It is likely that the trend for more magazines for the elderly will spread, and by finely cutting margins of profit, extend to those in lower income brackets who are now following trends set by those in the middle class of spending their money more freely in their last decades of life. The '50-Forward Club' undertook a huge promotion of its bi-monthly magazine *50 Forward* in 1989/90, and although about a third of the size of *Choice*, followed very closely in its image. Another recent magazine for older people is *Trust*, published on behalf of the Trustee Savings Bank Group. Because of the growing numbers of older people in the population, their economic power may have a powerful effect in changing the image of the elderly throughout society once they can be persuaded to adopt a new life-style.

In the course of an article appropriately titled 'Gold in Gray', Minkler (1989) presents many of the positive and the negative aspects of the growing awareness of the potential profitability of the grey-haired market. On the one hand, business interests can contribute to a meaningful old age by providing those goods and services that foster autonomy and make older people more part of the ordinary economy of the community. Advertisers can help to improve society's image of the elderly and give ageing people a better image of themselves. On the negative side, there is always the possibility that a misleading impression of the prosperity of the older section of the population may be conveyed, when in fact large numbers of older people are living in poverty and, as pointed out earlier, have no hope of benefiting from the goods and services that are offered to them. Such a misleading picture of the prosperity and homogeneity of the older population may adversely affect public policy in that governments may find increasing justification for cut-backs in the provision of health and social services for the considerable number of older people who are in real need of them.

## Popular humour

Jokes are a sensitive barometer of how people feel on certain issues, hence the popularity of sex jokes and lavatory humour in the aftermath of Victorian prudishness, and of black political jokes in repressive regimes. There have been a number of studies of how the perceived ridiculousness and nastiness of growing old is reflected in popular humour. Palmore's (1971) review of jokes about old people revealed that over half of them showed a highly negative attitude, and ageing women were the especial butt of aggressive humour. Richman (1977) compared jokes concerning the elderly with those about children, and found that whereas most of the jokes about children were appreciative, viewing them in a positive if 'quaint' light, most of the jokes about old people were definitely derogatory, ridiculing their physical decay, their growing stupidity, and the decline of their sexual powers. A few jokes were more complex, however, turning upon those who denigrate the elderly because their turn to be ridiculous would be coming in the course of time. Some jokes affirmed that some old people have a lot more life in them than is generally supposed, and in Fry's (1976) study of the psychodynamics of sexual humour, old men are portrayed as being absurd whatever they do, as they are seen either as sexless wrecks or over-sexed lechers. Davies (1977) analysed the content of 363 jokes about ageing and 187 jokes about death. Both categories showed an attitude of fear, and, as with other investigators, he found that ageist jokes were specially derogative of females.

Weber and Cameron (1978) have criticized the conclusions reached from these studies of popular humour as being too superficial, and indeed, they probably show more about the ambivalence of younger people's attitudes to the grandparent generation than sheer hostility and rejection.

There are two theories of the meaning and function of jokes that are worth considering, the disparagement theory and the incongruity model (Suls, 1976). It is easy to interpret jokes about old people in terms of disparagement theory, but unlike racist and sexist jokes, the younger people who make them know that they themselves will eventually be joining the group that is the butt of their humour. There is no way in which they can avoid taking on all the alleged characteristics of the stigmatized group except by dying young.

In the incongruity model, there is a necessary paradox to be perceived – that the crowing young man taking pride in his strength and virility will one day have to accept the decline that is in store for him. This is the riddle of the Sphinx that was posed to Oedipus – he who walks on two legs at noon, will hobble along on three in the evening.

That ageist jokes are particularly derogatory of women, is an example of the tragedy of the macho male's approach to sex, the knowledge that whoever he loves for her blooming, youthful charm, will be taken from him inevitably when she changes with age into someone he cannot approach in the same way.

In studying popular humour, greeting cards of various sorts are a valuable source of prevailing stereotypes. Birthday-card humour displays illustrative examples of aggressive ageism, often combined with sexism, and Itzen (1984) has found plenty of examples. There is, of course, the traditional mother-in-law joke; this aged female figure, ugly, stupid and domineering, has no counterpart in a father-in-law figure. The older woman represents what the young wife *will become* in the course of years, even though a man has specially chosen his spouse for her attractiveness and other good qualities. Birthday cards are particularly significant, as they remind people of the passing years and of the spectre of old age that looms ahead. Those designed to be sent to older relatives are typically sentimental and cheerful, reassuring the recipients that they don't look their age; it is those designed to be sent to contemporaries that contain crude jokes about the coming of old age with all its supposed horrors.

**Television**

There has been a lot of discussion of the negative image of older people depicted on American television. Undoubtedly the advertising industry has had a good deal to do with this, as in the past, though not so much nowadays, it is the younger age groups who have had the spending power, and must therefore be courted in TV programmes. Gerbner *et al.* (1980) carried out a study of American television with regard to the appearance of people who were apparently elderly, and concluded that 'Gross under-representations led viewers to believe that old people are a vanishing breed' (p. 37). They found that in prime-time TV drama, elderly men outnumbered elderly women by about three to one, and contrasted this with the showing of people in their twenties, among whom women outnumbered men because they are decorative and function in romantic character roles. Not only did men greatly outnumber women in the older age groups, but they appeared to age in appearance more slowly and show a greater enjoyment of life.

In view of this, the University of the Third Age in Cambridge, an independent and self-financing cultural and recreational body that caters mainly for retired people, undertook a research study to assess how British TV programmes presented images of 'the aged' (Lambert *et al.*, 1984). It was decided to monitor one whole week's TV broadcasting, and the output of all four channels over the period 23rd February–13th March 1983, taking BBC1 and Channel 4 during the first week, and ITV and BBC2 during the second week. They gave this task to fourteen monitors, only four of whom were under the age of 60, their main remit being to judge each programme as to whether it was fair or unfair in respect of the presentation of the image of the elderly.

Perhaps to the surprise of those who undertook this research, it was found that out of 487 programmes monitored only 22 could be described as being 'unfair' in the presentation of the elderly, although there were a further 34 in which the judges could not be sure. 'Elderly persons' were taken to be those judged by the monitors to be about 60 years old or older, and the question arises, of course, as to the degree to which monitors were agreed among themselves as to the identity of those they judged to be elderly. From the data they published there appears to have been no significant differences between the monitors.

What is of special interest is the degree to which programmes included or excluded elderly people. A breakdown of the 487 programmes monitored with regard to the presence/absence of elderly people is shown in Table 3.2.

While all types of programme had instances of elderly people being totally absent, their absence was particularly noticeable in the following: Plays, Serials, Soap Operas, Action/Adventure programmes, Situation Comedies, Schools and Education, Feature Films, Cartoons, Children's Programmes. They were normally totally absent from the last-named. Thus elderly persons appeared more frequently in programmes concerned with the news, current affairs and documentaries, and this was to be expected,

**Table 3.2** TV Programmes monitored for the age of people appearing

| Programmes | BBC1 | BBC2 | ITV | Channel 4 |
|---|---|---|---|---|
| With elderly persons | 116 (62%) | 40 (51%) | 86 (57%) | 43 (63%) |
| Without | 72 (38%) | 39 (49%) | 66 (43%) | 25 (37%) |

Data reprinted from *The Image of the Elderly on TV* with permission from The University of the Third Age in Cambridge.

as many prominent people in the world are elderly. As something like 20% of the population of the UK can now be classed as elderly, a fair presentation of group or crowd scenes would naturally present them in this proportion, or a little less, as perhaps they are less publicly visible. They were found to be roughly 10%–20% present in the groups shown. There were 1070 individual appearances, but in these the elderly were only *central figures* in only 292 cases; in the rest (72.7%) the elderly were marginal figures.

One striking feature of this inquiry relates to the sex of the elderly figures shown. Although women are in a significant majority among the elderly population, they were grossly under-represented in the TV programmes. Only 19.8% of the elderly figures were female, and they were seldom in central roles. This relates, of course, to the fact that it was in the news, documentary and current affairs programmes that older figures appeared more frequently, and there was a bias in favour of males as to the sex of politicians and other leading figures in the older age group.

The monitors found that it was possible to assess the social status of the elderly figures in 222 of the programmes, a total of 579 persons being so assessed. They found that the representation of the class composition of the elderly on television was as severely biased as the representation of their sex composition. Over four-fifths of those appearing belonged to the managerial and professional classes. This bias was less pronounced in fictional programmes where older working-class women had some significant role in popular soap operas such as Coronation Street. Taking into account both the sex and class distortions of the general presentations, the authors say 'The result can only be called a caricature of the real social world of the British elderly.' They make the point that 'an important reason why the elderly as

75

we know them are negligible in television appearance is *because* the successful elderly people who do figure there are not regarded as elderly in society. Thus, even when they are themselves biologically elderly, politicians and leaders do not represent the elderly as a social category.'

An attempt was made to rate the elderly on bi-polar characteristics such as wise/foolish, active/passive/, fit/infirm, where possible, dividing those rated into the three age categories 60–69, 70–79, 80+. There were 15 characteristics of this nature and on the first 14 the average number of rateable images was 469. On the 15th characteristic, however, there were only 47 images rated, and it stood out from the others by contrast. It was Sexually Active/Inactive (36/11). On the whole the findings of the rating of these characteristics were judged to be reasonably favourable, but the point has already been made that it was not the run-of-the-mill elderly who are shown on TV, but a rather superior class of people, and overwhelmingly male.

With regard to advertising, both ITV and Channel 4 were monitored. Although the elderly appeared rather seldom, when they were shown the image was fair and sympathetic. It may be that advertisers are now sensitive to the issues that have affected the launching of the magazines for retired people, as discussed earlier, and are anxious to appeal to this potentially lucrative and growing market.

In contrast to the earlier studies of the image of the elderly on American TV, this research found that British television presents older people in quite a favourable light, even in fictional programmes. The general criticism was that they appeared far less frequently than the proportion of the elderly in the present-day population justifies, and that those who are female, poor and of humble status get very little showing.

One interesting feature of British television is that in order to combat sexism and racism an equal number of male and female newscasters are now employed, and a number of coloured people. While newscasters may be female, all the women have to be relatively young and good-looking by contemporary standards. Male newscasters can have faces wrinkled with age, but no such wrinkled females are employed.

In the USA considerable attention was drawn to the image of the elderly on TV by social scientists in the late 1970s and 1980s, and there was considerable pressure to alter it (Davis and Davis,

1985). Some success has been achieved, and a more recent study of the portrayal of older adults in the context of family life showed that those over the age of 55 were represented generally more favourably than those approximating the mid-fifties (Dail, 1988). Again, however, the ratio of males to females was quite unbalanced (138 males to 55 females), and older women were depicted as being much more dependent and weak.

## CONCLUSION

We have discussed the stereotypes of the elderly as currently held by both professional and lay people, and it seems that although there is a growing liberalization of attitudes, we have a very long way to go yet in approaching anything like a reasonable view of ageing as an acceptable process in everyone's life. According to Freer (1988)

> Over the past fifteen years, particularly in the United States, there have been strenuous and welcome efforts to create a more informed view of ageing. These efforts have been strengthened by the growing research evidence from social gerontology, which, among other things, has provided a clearer understanding of ageing as distinct from disease. Unfortunately, most of what is written in the professional and lay press on topics related to the elderly makes it difficult to believe that these efforts have had any major impact (p. 3).

The reason why change is inevitably slow relates to the difference between thinking and feeling. People born in the earlier decades of this century were brought up by parents reared in the Victorian tradition, one aspect of which involved assigning to older people a very definitely sequestered role in society, especially with regard to their emotional and sexual lives. People may think in a quite rational and enlightened way on many of the issues that have been discussed, but emotional reactions are laid down in early childhood and determine attitudes in adult life, especially when these ageist attitudes are powerfully reinforced by literature, popular humour and folk-lore, and by the media, as discussed above. Adults born in later decades are, of course, the children, or the children's children of the Victorian-reared parents, and carry on the same tradition which accepts a double standard, not only with regard to relations between the sexes, but for relations between the generations.

It is not to be expected that professional people will be much different from lay people in their attitudes, for they have been subjected to the same formative influences in their development. The most they can do is to try to appreciate what the important issues are, and to realize what a great influence they may have in their professional capacity in furthering or retarding enlightened policies. Earlier in this chapter, evidence has been cited to the effect that emotional well-being has a very powerful effect on how people adapt to ageing, and provided that people have a satisfactory concept of themselves and are leading meaningful lives, they will adapt to whatever physical changes come with age and be no less contented and well-adjusted as the years progress.

The extent to which people's emotional well-being depends upon their sexuality is a matter about which we do not know a great deal because as a research area it is relatively new. There are some such as Wright (1985) who firmly declare that 'sexual activity is important for emotional and general well-being', and see it as an obvious component of a well-adjusted life-style in old age. It depends, of course, what is meant by 'sexual activity', a matter that will be explored throughout this book. Leviton (1973) brings forward impressive evidence that sexual activity in the later years of life preserves older people from depression and suicide, an important matter that has received very little attention in research so far. Leviton makes the point that there is an important need for the health professions to understand the relationship of sexuality with other aspects of therapy in treating the aged, and he contends that 'nearly all forms and types of loss can be related to the dysfunctioning of sexuality'.

It may be that Freer, as quoted above, is correct in judging that the efforts of social gerontologists have, so far, had little major impact. In the next chapter we will examine just what is being done, and what could be done, in the training of health-care professionals.

## REFERENCES

Becker, H. (1964) Personal change in adult life. *Sociometry*, 27, 40–53.
Berger, S.E. (1982) Sex in the literature of the Middle Ages: the

Fablieux, in Bullough, V.L. and Brundage, J. (eds) *Sexual Practices of the Medieval Church*, Prometheus Books, Buffalo, N.Y.

Brecher, E (1984), *Love, Sex, and Aging: A Consumer Union Report*, Little, Brown & Co, Boston.

Bury, M. (1988) Arguments about ageing: long life and its consequences, in Wells, N. and Freer, C. (eds) *The Ageing Population: Burden or Challenge?* pp. 17–31. The Macmillan Press, Basingstoke.

Coleman, P.G. (1983) Cognitive functioning and health, in Birren, J.E., Munnichs, J.M.A., Thomae, H. and Marios, M. (eds) *Aging: A Challenge to Science and Society, Vol. 3. Behavioral Sciences and Conclusions*, Oxford University Press, Oxford.

Chirikos, T.N. and Nestel, G. (1985) Longitudinal analysis of functional disabilities in older men. *J. Gerontol.*, 40, 426–433.

Comfort, A. (1990) *A Good Age*, Pan Books, London.

Cumming, E. (1963) Further thoughts on the theory of disengagement. *Int. Soc. Sci. J.*, 15, 377–393.

Cumming, E. and Henry, W. (1961) *Growing Old: The Process of Disengagement*, Basic Books, New York.

Dail, P.W. (1988) Prime-time television portrayals of older adults in the context of family life, *The Gerontologist*, 28, 700–706.

Dalton, K. (1978) *Once a Month*, Methuen, London.

Davies, L.J. (1977) Attitudes towards old age and aging as shown by humour, *The Gerontologist*, 17, 220–226.

Davis, R.H. and Davis, J.A. (1985) *TV's Image of the Elderly*, Lexington Books, Lexington, M.H.

De Beauvoir, S. (1972) *Old Age*, Penguin Books, Harmondsworth.

Dowd, J. (1975) Aging as exchange: a preface to theory. *J. Gerontol.*, 30, 584–594.

Featherstone, M. and Hepworth, M. (1984) Changing images of retirement, An analysis of representations of ageing in the popular magazine Retirement Choice, in Bromley, D.B. (ed.) *Gerontology: Social and Behavioural Perspectives*, pp. 219–224, Croom Helm, London.

Fisher, D. (1977) *Growing Old in America*, Oxford University Press, New York.

Ford, G. and Taylor, R. (1985) The elderly as underconsulters: a critical reappraisal, *J. Roy. Coll. Gen. Pract.*, 35, 244–247.

Freer, C. (1988) Old myths: frequent misconceptions about the elderly, in Wells, N. and Freer, C. (eds) *The Ageing Population: Burden or Challenge?* pp. 3–15. The Macmillan Press, Basingstoke.

Fries, J.F. (1980) Ageing, natural death and the compression of morbidity, *New Eng. J. Med.*, 303, 130–135.

Fry, W.F. (1976) Psychodynamics of sexual humour: sex and the elderly, *Med. Aspects Human Sex.*, 10, 140–141; 146–148.

Gerbner, G., Gross, L., Signorelli, N. and Morgan, M. (1980) Aging with television: Images in television drama and conceptions of social reality, *J. Communication*, 30, 37–47.

Gove, W. (1973) Sex, marital status and mortality, *Am. J. Sociol.* 79, 45.

Harris, L. (1975) *The Myth and Reality of Aging in America*,

The National Council on Aging, Washington, D.C.

Hochschild, A. (1975) Disengagement theory: a criticism and proposal. *Am. Sociol. Rev.*, 40, 553–569.

Itzin, C. (1984) The double jeapardy of ageism and sexism, in Bromley, D.B. (ed.), *Gerontology: Social and Behavioural Perspectives*, pp. 170–184, Croom Helm, London.

Khan, A.E. (ed.) (1970) *Joys and Sorrows: Reflections by Pablo Casals*, Simon & Schuster, New York.

Lambert, J., Laslett, P. and Clay, H. (1984) *The Image of the Elderly on TV*, University of the Third Age in Cambridge, Cambridge.

Leviton, D. (1973) The significance of sexuality as a deterrent to suicide among the aged, *Omega: J. Death Dying*, 4, 163–74.

Loughman, C. (1983) Eros and the elderly: a literary view. *The Gerontologist*, 20, 182–187.

Maddox, G.L. (1981) Measuring the wellbeing of older adults, in Somers, A.R. and Fabian, D.R. (eds) *The Geriatric Imperative: An Introduction to Gerontology and Clinical Geriatrics*, pp. 117–136, Appleton Century Crofts, New York.

Martel, M. (1968) Age–sex roles in American magazine fiction (1890–1955), in Neugarten, B. (ed.) *Middle Age and Aging* pp. 47–57, University of Chicago Press, Chicago.

Merriman, A. (1984) Social customs affecting the role of elderly women in Indian society in 1982, in Bromley, D.B. (ed.) *Gerontology: Social and Behavioural Perspectives*, pp. 151–162, Croom Helm, London.

Minkler, M (1989) Gold in gray: reflections on business' discovery of the elderly market, *The Gerontologist*, 29, 17–23.

Mossey, J.M. and Shapiro, E. (1982) Self-rated health: a predictor of mortality among the elderly, *Am. J. Pub. Health*, 72, 800–808.

Norman, A. (1987) *Aspects of Ageism: A Discussion Paper*, Centre for Policy on Ageing, London.

Palmore, E. (1971) Attitudes toward aging as shown by humor. *The Gerontologist*, 11, 181–186.

Petersen, D. and Karnes, E. (1976) Older people in adolescent literature, *The Gerontologist*, 16, 225–231.

Pfeiffer, E. and Davis, G.C. (1972) Determinants of sexual behavior in middle and old age, *J. Am. Geriat. Soc.*, 20, 151–158.

Pfeiffer, E., Verwoerdt, A. and Wang, H.S. (1968) Sexual behaviour in aged men and women, *Arch. gen. Psychiat.*, 19, 753–758.

Richman, J. (1977) The foolishness and wisdom of age: attitudes toward the elderly as reflected in jokes, *The Gerontologist*, 17, 210–219.

Seltzer, M. and Atchley, R.C. (1971), The concept of old: changing attitudes and stereotypes, *The Gerontologist*, 11, 226–230.

Suls, J. (1976) Cognitive disparagement theories of humour: a theoretical and empirical synthesis, in Chapman, A.J. and Foot, H.C. (eds) *It's a Funny Thing Humour*, pp. 41–45. Pergamon Press, Oxford.

Titmus, R.,M. (1959) *Essays on 'The Welfare State'*, Unwin University Books, London.

Victor, C.R. (1987) *Old Age in Modern Society*, Croom Helm, London.

Ward, R.A. (1954) *The Aging Experience*, Harper & Row, New York.

Weber, T. and Cameron, P. (1978) Comment: humor and aging – a response, *The Gerontologist*, 18, 73–76.

Wilkin, D. and Williams, E.I. (1986) Patterns of care for the elderly in general practice, *J. Roy. Coll. Gen. Pract.* 36, 567–570.

Wilson, J.B. (1982) Workload in a rural practice over the past eighteen years, *The Lancet*, 1, 733.

Wright, D. (1985), Sex and the elderly, *Nursing Mirror*, 161, 18–19.

# 4

# The role and training of
# health-care professionals

This chapter will attempt three things: (i) to describe very briefly
the nature of the training that is given in the chief professional
disciplines that are concerned with the care of the elderly; (ii) to
examine the extent to which such training includes the study of
gerontology and geriatrics, and gives practical experience of
working with older people; (iii) to consider the extent to which
the training, both pre and post-qualification, encompasses attention to more than sheer physical health and economic well-being,
and is concerned with aspects of the lives of older people that are
the subject of this book.

It is necessary to describe the outlines of the different professional trainings in order that those working in what has become a
field that is increasingly interdisciplinary should understand more
fully just what is the range of skills, status and competence of
their colleagues. Great changes have taken place in the latter half
of this century, and some people in the older professions are not
fully aware of precisely what role those in the newer disciplines
fulfil, and what changes are likely to take place in the future.
Quite obviously all specialists who deal with the health-care of
older people cannot be dealt with in this chapter for reasons
of space alone. For instance, the work of such specialists as
chiropodists and opticians is of special importance to elderly
people, but is not so relevant to the subject of this book, so need
not be discussed here.

## THE NEED TO RE-EXAMINE TRAINING IN THE
## HEALTH PROFESSIONS

All professional workers in health-care receive some instruction
and experience related to the needs of older people as part of

their training, but traditional practices are in need of some revision for two reasons. First, there is now a far greater proportion of the population who are elderly, and consequently the problems involved demand a greater degree of attention. A knowledge of geriatrics and social gerontology used to to be a very minor issue in the training courses, but it is now being asked whether much more attention should be paid to these subjects to prepare students adequately for the work they must do. Second, the nature of the problems encountered in later life has changed to some extent. The 'new old ' are not like those of previous generations in a number of ways. They have different expectations, different needs, and they are making new demands on professional workers.

Older social workers, nurses and doctors may remember how as students it was not uncommon to hear elderly people addressed in a jocose and patronizing manner simply because they were old, and therefore deemed to be a little dim-witted and grateful for any attention they might receive from professional care-givers. Most older people nowadays would resent such forms of address, and feel they had a right to receive what is their statutory entitlement without expressing special gratitude.

Regarding the percentage of older peeple in the community, it should be noted that at the turn of the century not more than 25% of the population in the developed countries survived beyond the age of 65, but nowadays about 70% of the population survive that age, and something over 30% of all deaths do not occur until after the age of 80 (Brody, 1988). In response to this radical change in the population structure, literature on the physical and emotional health of older people is expanding at a rapid rate, and it is difficult to keep up with all that is published. Much of what we thought we knew about the health, needs, abilities and attitudes of people in later life is in need of revision. In the past, such information was largely obtained from cross-sectional research, and has been shown to be unreliable by the newer longitudinal research studies that have followed up the same cohorts of people over a number of years (e.g. Busse, 1985; Coni *et al.*, 1984; Deeg, 1989; Evered and Whelan, 1988; Svanborg, 1985). It has been found that there are some very significant contrasts between the different generations as they age, due to the effects of their previous education, work experience, health record, and general lifestyle (Svanborg, 1988). As improved public health measures and physical medicine have lessened the seriousness of many acute illnesses such as pneumonia that used to be frequent killers of older people, so we are left with the chronic illnesses and, most importantly, the emotional disorders of later life that formerly were almost wholly unrecognized and neglected.

In summary, therefore, we may say that not only is there an increased need for professionals to be prepared to devote more time to the special needs that arise in later life, but that concentration on physical needs is now expanding to a study of emotional needs, and there is a growing recognition of the extent to which the two are interdependent.

This chapter will examine the extent to which the training courses for various professional specialisms include attention to geriatrics and social gerontology, and then consider the question of how that content relates to the emotional needs of older people, and how such education is concerned with affecting the *attitudes* of professional people, in addition to imparting factual *knowledge*. Considering the great variety of training courses provided for professional health-care givers, no comprehensive overview can be given in this chapter. Instead, some illustrative examples will be given, and then the general question of the principles that apply to all professional work will be discussed.

## NURSING AND HEALTH VISITING

Writing in 1991 it must be observed that the training of nurses is in a state of transition. The policy of 'Project 2000' is in the course of being implemented throughout the UK. Some Schools of Nursing are already operating the new system, others are preparing for it, and it is envisaged that it will not be finally implemented until 1994.

Briefly, Project 2000 involves the replacement of the old system of training recruits to the nursing profession solely as employed helps on the ward, by a three-year course of nurse education taking place in colleges of nursing and midwifery which will have links with colleges of higher education, and leads to a Diploma in Higher Education in nursing, and Registration to practise. The first 18 months will involve a Common Foundation

Programme providing a general introduction to nursing. This will be followed by a further 18 months in one of four branches, either (i) general nursing of adults, (ii) children's nursing, (iii) nursing the mentally ill, or (iv) nursing people with mental handicap.

The nursing care of the elderly comes first in the Common Foundation Programme, and then properly in branch (i). There is no branch devoted specifically to the care of the elderly as such, it being suggested by the Educational Policy Advisory Committee that specifying a particular age after which patients should receive care from an age group specialist would be unnecessary and tend to label people as 'elderly' (or 'geriatric') even though some people in their seventies are quite as fit, mentally and physically, as others in their fifties. Despite this obvious objection to a provision that might be described as ageist, the absence of a branch dealing with older people specifically can be criticised. For instance, older people react quite differently to some drugs and to illnesses; pneumonia will produce an acute illness in a young or middle-aged adult, with fever and delirium, but can affect an older person with no symptoms other than confusion, a symptom that sometimes gets a patient labelled as 'senile' and shunted into the chronic or psychiatric ward, although active treatment of the infection will restore lucidity. Harding (1990) comments that:

> Project 2000 recognizes that 'the task of improving the quality of life for older people with chronic illness and physical or mental impairment should be at the top of the agenda as amongst the greatest challenges for nursing in the future', yet sets no educational framework to meet these special needs (p. 8).

As to how far an educational framework can be laid down in the document in question is doubtful. To some extent it will depend on the traditions in the particular college of nursing and college of higher education. Harding goes on to cite 'A Strategy for Nursing' and notes that it advocates that all clinical practice should be founded on up-to-date information and research findings. She observes that conflicts may arise when current research-based theories filter through to the ground floor staff. The training and education given to the students may ensure that they know the theory, but they may find that the prevailing conditions of work prevent them form putting theory into practice. Staff may try to make the best use of the available resources in the prevailing circumstances, but finally get so disheartened that they leave the area of caring for the elderly.

### How far are nurses' attitudes to the elderly modified by training?

Here it must be emphasized that knowing something in theory, even if it is soundly based on research findings, does not necessarily mean that professionals will be willing to act on such knowledge, and nowhere is this more evident than in policies that relate to the emotional and sexual needs of older people. Where risks are involved, over-cautions and restrictive regimes that have the sanction of long tradition may be maintained in practice. Thus the trainee nurse may fear to be called to account for permitting too liberal a policy not obviously related to the direct physical needs of the patient.

The above tendency was well illustrated by a research project carried out by Glass *et al.* (1986) who studied seven nursing homes in one region of North Carolina. Some previous research studies (McContha and Stevenson, 1982; White, 1982) had indicated that the more knowledge nursing staff had of the facts of sexuality in later life, the more understanding and permissive they were in their professional practice. Glass and his colleagues set out to ascertain the extent of knowledge about sexuality in later life possessed by members of the staff of the nursing homes, and whether such knowledge was related to their attitudes to the elderly people in their care. They also studied whether socio-demographic characteristics such as age, marital status, general education, nursing education and religious denomination, were significantly related to both knowledge and education. Somewhat to their surprise they found that in this quite extensive study, the results were rather different from those coming from previous and smaller studies. The greater the extent of actual knowledge about sexuality in later life possessed by various members of the staff, the greater the degree of the restrictiveness of their attitudes towards the elderly. While the higher their general education, the more restrictive were their attitudes, this did not go for the level of *nursing education*, the latter being associated with greater understanding of the emotional needs of older people.

The above paradoxical findings can best be understood by a consideration of further datum from the study. Restrictiveness of attitude (and some members of the staff were characterized as being 'highly restrictive') was related to being in a supervisory and administrative position, such positions also going with having a higher level of general education, although not necessarily more nursing education. These findings are probably related to the question of professionals being rather cautious of taking risk. According to Comfort (1989):

> It's an old British custom that in the interests of military good order and discipline any institution, school, hospital, or home should be run like a good gaol – people in it should be clean, tidy, idle and not called on to make choices. Older people in Britain are spared the excesses of the American nursing home racket; there fit people are kept in bed because the owners get higher subventions for the bedridden. Here they may be kept unnecessarily in bed because it's tidier like that. . . . Sexuality is a particular bugbear of the British institution. It's only recently that homes (some of them) ceased to separate married couples, and any formation of new relationships may still cause acute administrative embarrassment (p. 120).

Norman (1987) has argued that the emotional health and dignity of older people are in danger of being undermined by professionals in the Health Service being too concerned to protect them from 'risk', but that some element of risk is inseparable from self-determination. Nursing staff sometimes regard elderly patients rather as children in their care, and to be protected from their own wayward inclinations and behaviour. The question arises – what are the real emotional needs of people in later life? Do they really need a love-life, or are they better off reconciled to the conventional idea that all that sort of thing is redundant after middle-age? Passive, sexless types of patient are certainly more convenient to handle and, apart from being less vulnerable to any possible risks to themselves, pose no risks to their carers getting into trouble from figures in authority censoring them for their liberal policies of management.

All these issues need to be fully explored in the training of nurses. It is not enough to give them simple instruction; they have to be encouraged to examine their own personal attitudes to older people of both sexes. Among female nurses a certain degree of feminist protest may make them all too ready to protect their elderly female patients from what they may regard as emotional and sexual exploitation by male patients, and such matters need to be examined.

It should be considered whether women old enough to be the nurses' grandmothers are really in need of such solicitous protection, or whether, in the words of Kellett (1989), discussing the sexuality of older people, 'They should make their own decisions' with regard to emotional involvements.

### Controversy in the nursing journals

There has been considerable discussion in the nursing journals over the past decade, both in the UK and the USA, about nurses' roles in inhibiting or facilitating the expression of sexuality among older patients under their care, both at home and in institutions. Thus some writers such as Griggs (1978) and McCarthy (1979) are of the opinion that some professionals have gone too far in encouraging elderly people to express their sexuality, when they were quite content with celibacy. It may be noted that McCarthy uses the unfortunate term 'geriatric sexuality', as do some other American writers when they mean love-making between older people. Others, such as Griffiths (1988) and Wright (1985), regard love-making between older people as positively enriching their lives, and something that the nursing profession should study how best to facilitate.

It is admitted that the expression of sexuality in a hospital or similar setting may cause great embarrassment to the nursing staff. Thus Emily Griffiths, a staff nurse, relates how, when seeking to comfort an elderly man, she held his hand and asked if she could do anything for him; he replied by seriously suggesting that she should get into bed with him. She goes on to observe that:

There are two main reasons why sexuality in the elderly is difficult to discuss. First, nurses historically have not been trained to cope with sexuality. Their sexuality is 'suppressed and repressed', with the aim of 'purity' and 'asexuality', and they suffer from sexism and stereotyping at work. But if nurses are not aware of their own attitudes, beliefs and values, they will not be able to help others (Griffiths, 1988, p. 34).

The second reason for embarrassment in discussing the expression of sexuality among older people that she gives relates to the ageism of a youth-oriented society, making it difficult for older people to verbalize the nature of their emotional feelings for fear of being seen as depraved and lecherous. She states that while there is a considerable literature on counselling following medical and surgical interventions, she could find none referring to patients' need for sexual expression, only some on 'inappropriate sexual behaviour in residential homes'.

Damrosch (1984) questions whether the taboo on facing the reality of sexuality among older people is now as strong as many writers assume. She reports on her study involving the attitudes of 114 students enrolled in a Master of Science nursing programme. It transpired that their image of a (hypothetical) 68-year-old woman was positively enhanced by the information that the woman was sexually active, either married or unmarried. When the account of this hypothetical woman was presented without the added information that she was sexually active, she was perceived as less well-adjusted, mentally alert, healthy, etc. The one negative thing that the sexually active image conveyed to these nursing students was that such a woman would be less popular with hospital staff! It may be, therefore, that the rising generation of nursing students are less biased against the concept of sexually active elderly people than we have come to assume. Damrosch mentions that the students in her study had already been exposed to some educative influences to liberalize their attitudes to the elderly.

Wright (1985) states that it is now generally accepted that sexual activity is 'important for emotional and general well-being'. She states that although the nursing and social work press are beginning to question traditional attitudes to sexuality in the elderly, 'Sexuality is not even acknowledged or catered for.' How far that is still true in the nursing profession is questionable. She goes on to state:

> The literature suggests that health workers need to look at their own sexuality and also gain some understanding of the subject. Perhaps we then can cater for the client's needs. I

think that this is particularly important for nurses. We claim to be concerned with the whole individual and yet we ignore an essential part of that individual's life. Some of the issues in this article have great implications for health educators and workers. The elderly often get a rough deal; perhaps we can start improving the situation by acknowledging their sexuality (Wright, 1985).

Reviewing these various publications, it seems that the nursing profession is in a state of transition, and what evidence we have about the current attitudes of young and not-so-young people towards the emotional lives of the elderly, and how far sexuality, conceived of as a genital phenomenon, needs to be expressed, is somewhat contradictory. It is to be hoped that in training programmes for nurses these issues will be explored fully and frankly. It is not merely a question of being permissive in allowing people the facilities for fostering affectionate relationships in later life in the manner they choose, despite the constraints of their impaired health and the demands of a hospital or similar regime. Nurses should expect to play a positive role in assisting elderly people to get the best out of life. This point is put very forcefully by Katzin (1990) in an article that begins by discussing how patients can be advised in techniques to minimize the handicaps of three disabilities (chronic obstructive pulmonary disease, arthritis, and diabetes) in enjoying their sex-lives, and then goes on to tackle the whole question of the nurse's general role as health counsellor in facilitating their elderly patients' love relationships, with due tact and sensitivity.

## CLINICAL PSYCHOLOGY

### The founding of the profession

Clinical psychology, as an independent discipline, is a relatively new profession in the UK, in contrast to the USA, where a professional organization was founded in 1917, so it will be useful to describe it briefly before discussing its services to the elderly. In Britain up until the 1940s there were a number of so-called clinical psychologists attached to psychiatric hospitals and clinics, but they had had little professional training, and what training they had received was generally in the educational field and in Child Guidance clinics. The public, and indeed many psychiatrists in past times, erroneously assumed that a university graduate in psychology had some special competence in dealing with clinical problems, but this was hardly the case. Studies in a university degree course were necessarily theoretical in orientation, and, unlike a medical course, gave no professional training. so they might have little relevance to the clinical field.

Clinical psychology, as a distinct and properly qualified profession in the UK, began to be organized in the 1940s, as described by Davidson (1953), and de Monchaux and Kier (1961). The psychologists' professional society, the British Psychological Society (BPS), originally founded under that name in 1906, liaised with the educational services and founded the 'Committee of Professional Psychologists: Mental Health' in 1943, and was actively concerned to promote this new profession. What was lacking, of course, was a proper scheme of university-based training similar to that which is given to medical students. A clinical postgraduate course for psychologists was first introduced by the initiative of a psychiatrist, Professor Aubrey Lewis, at the Institute of Psychiatry, London University, in the department of the psychologist Hans Eysenck, and ran in conjunction with the Maudsley and Bethlem Hospitals. The course was started in 1947 and provided a 13-month clinical training, for which a Diploma was awarded. Other training schemes began at the Crichton Royal Hospital and the Tavistock Institute, but they could not confer university diplomas.

In those early days, clinical psychologists' concern with the elderly was largely in the assessment of cognitive deterioration, but more and more their work involved rehabilitation. However, with the growth of the behaviour therapy movement, which was pioneered in the UK by Eysenck and his colleagues (Eysenck, 1958), and in the USA by Skinner and his associates (Skinner and Lindsley, 1953), clinical psychologists began to be heavily involved in the treatment process as independent professionals, often acting in association with psychiatrists and other medical doctors, but not under the control of the latter as were paramedical therapists.

The further development of the profession is well described by Liddell (1983). Clinical psychologists now have a professional training which is normally of three years' duration after graduation in an honours degree in psychology. This training is achieved through two alternative channels. It may be based on a university or polytechnic academic department of psychology, with placements for practical work in clinics, hospitals, or working in the community, and this postgraduate course leads to the award of an MSc or PhD degree. Alternatively, the course may consist of supervised in-service training, the students studying for the award of the Clinical Diploma of the British Psychological Society. The usual career grade of clinical psychologists is the Senior Psychologist, and to reach this psychologists have normally done about five years postgraduate training. There are, of course, higher grades attainable after more extensive experience.

In 1972 a sub-committee of the Standing Mental Health Advisory Committee was established 'To consider the role of psychologists in the Health Services' (Trethowan, 1977). They were mainly concerned with what clinical psychologists did, and might do, in the National Health Service, but considered also the work of educational and some other psychologists. In 1962 there had been 198 people in the new profession of clinical psychology in England and Wales, and by 1973 this number had grown to only 585, a very small increase in view of the demand that the Trethowan Committee identified. It was noted that the profession had developed in close association with psychiatry, and most of the work had been in the field of mental illness and mental handicap. The Report of the Trethowan Committee stated that:

> There has, however, been a steady change in the nature of the contribution made by psychologists to the treatment of patients. In former times their role consisted largely of undertaking routine psychological measurements, such as intelligence testing at the request of psychiatrists and other doctors, and represented in effect an ancillary service to the medical profession. Recent years have seen a substantial expansion in the body of psychological knowledge accompanied by the development of new techniques which have major implications for treatment (Trethowan, 1977, p. 2).

From the evidence they gathered the Committee estimated that clinical psychologists were spending about 45% of their time in 'treatment and rehabilitation'.

## Clinical Psychology and the elderly

During the 1970s when the future of clinical psychology was being debated, it was seldom noted how the population structure was altering so that there was a greatly growing need for psychologists to give their services in the care of the elderly. The Trethowan Committee noted that:

> We were told that the involvement of psychologists in the clinical management of geriatric patients is at present minimal or non-existent. The British Geriatric Association told us that they would welcome more participation by psychologists in this field, in particular in helping to develop a therapeutic milieu in wards and day hospitals, and in developing programmes to help elderly people in adjusting to their failing functions (Trethowan, 1977, p. 8).

In response to this need a group of clinical psychologists who were working with elderly people formed an unofficial association in 1980 which was later called the Psychologists' Special Interest Group in the Elderly, (PSIGE) and became officially affiliated with the Division of Clinical Psychology of the BPS. This group has now grown considerably in size and numbers about 230 members, all of them working in some capacity with elderly people in a great variety of settings. The PSIGE publishes a substantial quarterly Newsletter.

There is still a wide variation in the number of hours devoted to teaching about the care of the elderly in different training schemes for clinical psychologists. Andrew Norris (reported by Candy, 1990) conducted a survey of different training courses in 1986 and found that while one included 66 hours in a three-year course, at the other extreme, another provided only 15 hours teaching in a course of similar length. The average number of teaching hours devoted to the elderly was 28.3, and clinical placements with the elderly averaged 4.8 months. Only 24% of the courses surveyed had a compulsory placement with the elderly in the core component. Clinical psychologists qualifying by in-service placements, and sitting the BPS Diploma examination, do not have to have a placement in work with the elderly. Although they can have such a placement as an option if they wish it, early in their careers they can decide to avoid work with the elderly.

## The attitudes of clinical psychologists to older people

As a professional discipline, clinical psychology is especially concerned with people's emotional lives, and exhibits a significant difference from medicine. The latter is concerned primarily with geriatrics, and relates to ageing in terms of the medical model, whereas psychology is concerned with ageing more in terms of gerontology, the study of normal function and personal adjustment in ageing. The medical profession has done most important work in elucidating the physiological changes in the sexual function with ageing, and developing therapeutic procedures, much of their work being referred to in the present book. On the other hand, psychologists, taking a different approach, have been rather more influential in devising programmes of behavioural therapy. In fact, medical doctors have generally worked in sex therapy together with psychologists and therapists in other therapeutic disciplines, as is apparent from the various books that draw contributions from more than one discipline. Joint publications often have a medical and a non-medical author (e.g. Butler and Lewis, 1988; Gillan and Gillan, 1976; Greengross and Greengross, 1989; Masters and Johnson, 1966, 1970).

As far as training is concerned, clinical psychologists have shown themselves to be fairly liberal-minded towards the sexual lives of older people. This may relate, to some degree, to the fact that clinical psychology is such a new profession, and has not inherited the Victorian legacy of repressive attitudes towards ageing and sexuality that affected the older professions of nursing and medicine in the past. Arentewicz and Schmidt (1983) investigated the reactions of different professional groups to training that involved sex therapy. They found that nurses and medical doctors had difficulty in accepting that therapy consisted of treating relationships rather than sick patients. Trainees in other professional backgrounds, such as clinical psychologists and social workers, showed less of this bias of the medical model.

Although clinical psychologists may be fairly liberal in their views, they are not much different, as students, from those in other disciplines in what amounts to a fear of dealing with elderly people. An anonymous Course Co-ordinator at a polytechnic makes the following abservations about introducing the topic of the care of older people to third year psychology students:

> One thing I'm absolutely certain of is that there is absolutely no point in starting to teach about the elderly till the trainees' own fears have been dealt with. I had the sad experience of giving a workshop to *third year* clinical psychology trainees and very quickly it became very clear to me and the colleague I brought with me that a great majority of them were petrified by the elderly.... The level of anxiety was palpable ... only one in twelve 'thinking about' working with the elderly (C.C., 1990, p. 18).

So far there has been very little reported work investigating the attitudes of clinical psychologists to the sexuality of older people. Simpson (1984) investigated the attitudes towards older people of clinical psychologists compared with those of medical students, and concluded that the former group were less ageist than the latter. He suggested that 'The slightly unfavourable view of the elderly, especially by some of the medical students, results from a perceived greater likelihood of old people behaving in ways that are viewed as slightly unpleasant.' He did not inquire specifically about sexual behaviour, and it is possible that the differences he found were rather specific to the groups he studied. A review of the file of the past ten years of the Newsletter of the PSIGE does not show any discussion of the question of clinical psychologists being concerned about their roles in inhibiting or facilitating the expression of sexuality among the elderly people under their care. This contrasts with the concern of the nursing profession, as shown in their journals discussed above. This lack of discussion may be interpreted either as psychologists being quite open-minded on the issue, so that no controversy arises, or that the issue is deemed too unimportant in a profession that is greatly understaffed and overstretched in trying to cope with rehabilitation after strokes, over-stressed families, and other problems of a basic nature that are perceived as having priority. One might have thought that clinical psychologists, in their efforts to improve the quality of life for elderly people under their care, would have been concerned with questions of sexual fulfilment and, for instance, the problems that arise because of the lack of privacy in many residential homes. However, there is little evidence of this in their published literature.

## MEDICINE

Medicine is a very well-established profession, and it is therefore unnecessary to describe the nature of medical training courses, which have not changed basically for a long time, and are unlikely to change much in the future. Instead, it may be helpful to consider very briefly the component of such courses that is concerned with the care of older people. Here there have been changes, and further changes may be expected in the future as the size of the elderly population increases.

The British Medical Association (1976) produced a report on the care of the elderly, recommending that each medical school should have an academic unit 'to provide authoritative undergraduate and postgraduate teaching in the clinical problems of old people, together with some knowledge of gerontology and of the administrative structure of services for the aged'. It should be noted that *gerontology* was mentioned, for among medical doctors their services to the elderly are generally considered exclusively in terms of *geriatric medicine*. In practice, however, the GP is concerned with more than 'the clinical, preventive, remedial and social aspects of illness in the elderly', which is the definition of geriatric medicine given by the BMA. Whether he or she likes it or not, the GP is consulted by older people concerned with the quality of the lives they are leading. They are often vague about the nature of their problem; they may call it insomnia, anxiety, depression, indigestion or a magnification of the 101 problems to which we are all subject, but hardly notice when we are leading a full and rewarding life. The unfortunate GP tends to reach for the prescription pad and treat the complaint symptomatically, handing out sleeping pills, anxiolytics, antidepressives, palliative medicines for indigestion, etc., while ruminating that what is really wrong with such patients is that they are 'old'. Geriatric medicine has no remedy for being 'old'.

Social gerontology has made the problems associated with ageing rather more comprehensible. As noted in the Chapter 3, it is not just the objectively diagnosed health that is of primary importance, but the 'subjectively perceived well-being' (Mossey and Shapiro, 1982), and this is largely a function of the elderly person's emotional status. Fortunately, in courses labelled geriatric medicine a certain amount of gerontology is included, but such courses vary a very great deal according to the medical school, both as to the amount taught and the method and content of teaching.

## The studies of Smith and Williams

In 1981 Smith and Williams (1983) sent a questionnaire to the deans and teachers of geriatric medicine at all 30 of the clinical medical schools in the UK. The replies indicated that in all but two there was some teaching of geriatric medicine, but it varied greatly in amount between schools, 10 of them providing 3–50 hours teaching, and three schools had as many as 151–171 hours. They reported that 'In most schools all medical students receive teaching in geriatric medicine but in some. . . . only a proportion (18–50%) of students have clinical teaching in the subject and this is usually during general medical training' (p.2). They noted that formal teaching in gerontology was included in the first or second year of seven medical schools, a Department of Geriatric Medicine generally being involved. The fact that some medical students did not get a compulsory and complete coverage of the subject was not in line with the World Health Organization recommendation that *all* should have in their curricula the study of human development and ageing in all its aspects, including the psychological, epidemiological and sociological (WHO,1974). That the position at that time was less than ideal in view of the facts of the rapidly changing population structure, must be considered in the light of the great improvements that were being introduced. In 1975 an average of only 35 hours of teaching was provided (Nuffield Trust, 1977), but by 1981 the average had risen to 69 hours, as determined by Smith and Williams.

The World Health Organization produced a later report 'Learning objectives in gerontology and geriatric medicine' (WHO, 1982) one table of which is reproduced here in Table 4.1.

Stout (1985) discusses this and reproduces a number of schemes of the educational objectives of various medical schools in the UK and the USA. It is instructive to consider these schemes in terms of the relative emphasis they give to sheerly disease-

**Table 4.1** Teaching objectives for undergraduate teaching in gerontology

---

1. To develop an understanding of the complete life cycle: development, maturation and ageing, one part of which gradually merges into the next.
2. To demonstrate the importance of knowledge of the normal ageing processes, for the purposes of differentiation between them and illness in old age.
3. To produce an understanding that the normal adult person undergoes changes beyond the standard '25-year-old, 70-kg male'.
4. To ensure a background knowledge of reduced adaptability during ageing, which is a basis for the pathenogensis of the altered disease manifestation of the aged.

---

Source: World Health Organization (1982) *Teaching Gerontology and Geriatric Medicine*: Report on a workshop, Edinburgh 5–7 April, WHO publication ICP/ADR 045 (2).

orientated geriatric medicine, compared with the newer emphasis on relating medicine to healthy ageing, and enhancing the fulfilment of life at all ages.

In 1986 Smith and Williams (1988) repeated their survey, sending out questionnaires to all the medical schools concerning their teaching of geriatric medicine. Although there had been a small increase in the hours spent in teaching the subject, in two schools only a proportion of medical students received such instruction as it was not compulsory. Only 39% of the schools were teaching formal gerontology. On the whole, the position had not changed much in the five years that had elapsed, and Smith and Williams concluded their report by recommending that 'The schools who do not teach the subject formally or give inappropriately little time to it, should be reconsideriing their curriculum to meet the needs of the population of the 21st century' (p. 500).

## A qualitative survey

Following the two surveys of Smith and Williamson, Gibson (1990) circulated all the deans of medical schools and faculties of medicine, explaining that information on the teaching of gerontology/geriatric medicine was required for the present book concerned with the emotional and sexual lives of older people. No questionnaire was used, as in the case of the Smith and Williams studies, for the object was to present an open-ended request, and let the medical schools reply in their own way, only an impressionistic rather than a statistical summary of the position being required. A great wealth of material was provided by the medical schools, and due justice cannot be done to it here. Some respondents replied with quite lengthy letters, and enclosed schemes of teaching, and other relevant material. It was evident that, as shown by the earlier surveys, a great variety of approach, both quantitatively and qualitatively, existed in the various professional courses. Extracts from the letters of six of the respondents will suffice to illustrate the most important points.

One Consultant Physician in a Department of Medicine for the Elderly wrote, 'I am afraid the teaching of Medicine of Old Age . . . is very limited at the moment and (students) only spend a week with us during their final medical firms. . . . We are in the process of reorganising the course and I hope, starting from next year, that we will run an integrated course with the Department of General Practice, Community Medicine and Psychiatry lasting 24 weeks.' Another respondent, a Professor of Geriatric medicine, indicated that since 1974 students had had 40 hours of geriatric medicine in the 3rd (i.e. 1st clinical) year of the course, and kindly enclosed a teaching programme. He wrote, 'As you will see, the emphasis in the course is very largely on the medical aspects of old age, rather than on the topics you mention.'

In contrast, some respondents indicated that the emotional and sexual lives of older people were given special attention in the teaching course. In one university medical school they are concerned to break down the traditional barrier between pre-clinical and clinical training, and include a course in social gerontology preclinically, giving the students attachments to general practitioners during which they 'adopt' a family which contains elderly or disabled people. The professor there writes 'At an early stage in the course several hours of teaching are devoted to "Medical Sexology", and I know that in these lectures reference is made to the sexual lives of older people.' A number of medical schools are introducing a greater interdisciplinary approach in the teaching of social gerontology; from one such school the professor makes the point that their object is not to train 'embryonic consultant geriatricians', but to equip the students

with the skills and attitudes necessary to care for elderly people. One particular lecture is given by an elderly lady who describes the sexual attitudes as they were when she was a girl and goes on to describe how her own sexuality (and that of her husband) evolved over the years. This lecture provides very pertinent insights for the young students.

The great wealth of information that modern research has given the medical profession about the disease processes in later life has presented a certain dilemma in teaching: how to balance the direction of students' studies between the diagnostic aspects of medicine and the treatment of various pathological conditions that afflict a small minority of older people, and a necessary appreciation of the nature of the physical and emotional well-being of the normal majority who need some attention from doctors in their role of counsellors and specialist advisors. In the past, geriatric medicine over-emphasized the former aspect of the doctor's role. A consultant geriatrician writes:

> The essence as I see it of teaching geriatric medicine is to emphasise not only diagnostic and investigative aspects of disease but to emphasise the emotional aspect and the physical and mental consequences of disabling disease in old age. . . . Another major component of the undergraduate course is trying to teach the skills of communicating with elderly people who have got problems with communication and this surely has a lesson for dealing with older people in general.

One consequence of familiarizing students with the most serious pathological conditions that occur in old age, necessary though it is, is that they may get a biased view and fail to appreciate how basically healthy and potentially vigorous most elderly people are, given the right social and personal environment and positive psychological orientation. Another Professor of Geriatric Medicine mentions this, and how he tries to overcome such bias. He writes:

> The clinical practice of our department is that we take responsibility for the frailest and most disabled of the elderly patients in the hospital, deliberately seeking out those with the most complex multiple disability. . . . There is, of course, a real risk that this will give a distorted view of normal ageing, emphasising all the dreadful things that can happen, and leading the student to forget the fact that most elderly people are relatively untroubled by such problems. This is an important

issue which we address with our students in my introductory seminar.

## The attitudes of medical students

Some concern has been expressed, both in the UK and the USA, about the attitudes of medical students to their patients, both in relation to ageing itself and concerning sexual matters. Diseker and Michielutte (1981) suggest that, for American students at least, the original selection process is biased in favour of non-empathic students, and Kramer, Ber and Moor (1989) state that a process of 'dehumanization' takes place as students proceed through their medical studies. They state that while 'Empathic listening to patients, responding to their emotional needs, and expressing supportive caring are the main components of an empathic approach, unfortunately these are often considered a waste of time in the hospital setting, and are discouraged by clinical tutors' (p. 168).

All too often medical textbooks appear to inculcate in students an assumption that they can safely ignore any lingering sexual needs that older prople may have. Thus in *Medicine in Old Age* (British Medical Association, 1985), there are 22 articles which appear to take this assumption for granted when sexuality is relevant to what is being discussed: for example, the possible side effects of impotence attendant on the prescription of certain drugs for the elderly (as discussed in Chapter 1) are not even mentioned. Hormone replacement therapy is mentioned – but not for the most obvious use that some post-menopausal women require it. Medical students' negative assumptions about the elderly may be reinforced by such textbooks.

There have been attempts to modify the attitudes of medical students towards the elderly, such as that of Smith and Wattis (1989), but they do not appear to have been very effective. More successful have been the attempts to modify students' attitudes towards sexuality in general. Stanley (1978) cites a number of studies of this nature, and describes a programme that she and her colleagues initiated at St George's Hospital in London. Basically the programme consisted of showing the students a series of 17 short films in six sessions, dealing very explicitly with various sexual situations, and discussing the students' own reactions in seminars. The sessions referred to: (i) ordinary heterosexual relations; (ii) masturbation; (iii) homosexuality; (iv) situations involving lovemaking in pregnancy, with physical handicap, and between 'older' people; (v) body-communication with autistic children; (vi) sex therapy. According to the later seminar discussions and a questionnaire, the students' attitudes appeared to have been modified in a positive direction, and it emerged that:

> Encouraging numbers felt that their attitudes had changed towards greater acceptance and understanding about each topic in the questionnaire, particularly in relation to sexuality in the elderly and physically handicapped (p. 443).

We are told that in the lovemaking scene between the couple representing the 'elderly', the man was aged 63 and the woman 50! This is hardly what most people would consider to be 'elderly'. The man was 13 years older than the women, and one wonders what the students' reactions would have been if the couple had both been in their 70s, or the woman had been considerably older than the man. Perhaps the intention was to let the students down lightly without too great a transgression of traditional prejudices.

Apart from Stanley's study, and those she cites in her paper, there have been various other projects to investigate and to modify the attitudes of medical students to sexuality and to the elderly (Damrosch and Fishman, 1985; Davies, 1987; Hawton, 1979; Lamberti and Chapel, 1977; Vollmer and Wells, 1988). It would seem that this is a part of medical education that should not be neglected at the undergraduate level, although there is plenty of opportunity to enlarge upon it in postgraduate courses, as will be mentioned later. However, apart from such special projects, the best approach would obviously be to pay attention to the students' attitudes during the whole course of their education in their role of caring for the elderly, as appears to be the case in some of the medical schools cited.

## SOCIAL WORK

The profession of social work has its history in the charitable field, as well as in the Poor Law, and the modern concept of the citizen, adult or child, being entitled to social welfare as of right, goes quite against a long tradition of Utilitarian social philosophy, as expressed by such writers as Joseph Townsend, and Thomas Malthus, and the Social Darwinism of Herbert Spencer. The thesis of the present book is that elderly people are entitled to expect services from professional people that not only ensure minimal standards of nutrition, health, and adequate housing, but contribute to their general emotional well-being and enjoyment of life *according to their own personal standards*. This may not meet with unqualified approval from all social workers. The attitudes inherent in Utilitarianism and Social Darwinism no longer dominate social welfare policies, but somewhat similar attitudes still persist, and deserve to be discussed. Earlier, in the section describing training for the nursing profession, writers were quoted (e.g. Griggs, 1978; McCarthy, 1979) who rather deplored the positive encouragement that was being given in some quarters to elderly people to believe that they were entitled to expect a satisfying love-life, whatever their marital status and sexual preferences. How far such a point of view is expressed in the training of social workers needs to be examined.

Training for the social work profession, like the nursing profession, is currently in the process of transition. Since 1987 two social work qualifications have been recognized throughout the UK: the Certificate in Social Service (CSS) and the Certificate of Qualification in Social Work (CQSW). These are awarded by a national body, the Central Council for Education and Training in Social Work (CCETSW). This Council is now phasing out, over the next five years, training for these two qualifications, and replacing them with a new qualification, the Diploma in Social Work (Dip.SW).

### The new Diploma in Social Work

Details of the scheme for introducing the new Diploma are given in *Paper 30*, a publication of the award-giving body (CCETSW, 1989). There will be no more recruitment for the courses leading to the two social work Certificates mentioned above after 1994.

The courses for the DipSW will last at least two years; initially they will be either employment-based or college-based, and eventually it is hoped that through a system of credit accumulation and transfer this distinction will become less absolute. The current output of qualified social workers is about 4,200 a year, and according to the CCETSW *Paper 30* this is already inadequate and they plan to raise it to 5,000 a year. How these extra social workers will be deployed is not stated, but in view of the steadily changing age structure of the population, presumably the balance of services to the younger/older sections of the community is being considered.

## The attitudes of social workers towards older people

While in the training provided for the nursing and medical professions serious and deliberate attention has been given to the examination of students' attitudes to older people in general, and to their emotional and sexual lives, there is not a great deal of evidence that such concern is shown in relation to trainee social workers. In *Paper 30* under the heading of 'The Values of Social Work', it is stated that qualifying social workers must be able to:
- demonstrate an awareness of both individual and institutional racism and ways to combat both through anti-racist practice
- develop an understanding of gender issues and demonstrate anti-sexism in social work practice (CCETSW, 1990, p. 16).

While it is entirely laudable that awareness of the issues of racism and sexism should be part of the training of social workers, it is perhaps surprising that ageism is not mentioned specifically as well, as certain prejudices against older people, particularly in relation to the conduct of residential homes, has long been a feature of the care of the elderly (Comfort, 1989; Eastman, 1987; McCartney *et al.*, 1987; Norman, 1987). Stout (1985) points out that, 'Attitudes towards the elderly, of both the population as a whole and of some members of the health professions are sometimes unhelpful and negative'. No doubt this question comes in for a good deal of discussion in some training courses, but it does not feature prominently in the journals associated with the social work profession. Looking back in the file of *Community Care*, the social workers' main journal, references to older people principally concern issues of housing, dementia, hypothermia, home care services, and other bread and butter issues. There is little evidence that it is recognized that 'man cannot live by bread alone', or that social workers are trying to live up to the avowed aim of contributing to the quality of the majority of their clients' lives, irrespective of their age. Considering the many cases of extreme and tragic need for help on the part of some elderly people and their carers, so movingly related by writers such as Eastman (1984), it is not surprising that these cases are given a good deal of prominence in the social work journals; but there might be more debate about the emotional needs of older people. There are exceptions. Skinner (1988), in the above mentioned journal, makes quite a forceful plea for the sexual needs of older people to considered by social workers and the staff of residential homes, and argues that:

> It is important to be aware that a satisfactory sexual relationship is important for most people's well being at any age. In the elderly the increased need for love, self-esteem and for close human contact give sexuality an enhanced value.... Professional staff need to be aware of compounding the problem through projecting their own taboos by, for instance, discouraging developing liaisons (p. 25).

Like the clinical psychologists, the social workers also have a special interest group for those concerned with working with older people, (SIGA), and this might be expected to explore the relevant issues in greater depth than the profession as a whole. They were given a talk on *Sexuality in Later Life* by Dr Mary Davies (McKenzie, 1988), but this appears to have been a somewhat unusual occurrence. It should be noted that both Dr Skinner and Dr Davies, whose contributions are noted above, are clinical psychologists. Dr Simon Biggs, another psychologist, who is a social work education advisor to the CCETSW, has produced an excellent manual of exercises designed to explore the attitudes of social workers to the elderly, (Biggs, 1989). More might be done along these lines touching more sensitive areas in which people have embarrassment in relating to older clients.

In a personal communication, a very senior social worker associated with their Special Interest Group on Ageing, writes:

> I recall no mention of the sexual lives of older people on my professional course, and my colleagues in my area office... report the same of their training courses.... The absence of expertise is reflected in books on social work with older people. We rely possibly on organisations like Relate and their

counselling skills. We are only just beginning to tackle principles and procedures in Social Service Departments about sexual abuse of older people. The residential sector of social work may have more to say about sexual expression than fieldworkers like myself.

Maybe I am being unfair on the social work profession, and it would be gratifying to learn through your reseach whether there are social workers having lively discussions. Let's hope that in the assessment of older people's needs with the community care plans of 1991 we are required to tackle their sexual needs.

## POSTGRADUATE AND INTERDISCIPLINARY TRAINING COURSES

The Griffiths Report observes that health-care professionals in every discipline and all administrative staff need training that not only enables them properly to fulfil their own roles in relation to the elderly, but to understand the contribution of other professionals. It states:

> Insularity among individual professional groups can lead to failures of communication and inability to recognise both needs and options for meeting them. The need for effective collaboration in training matters at the local level to tackle this should be addressed to all authorities, both during the implementation period and as an on-going task (Griffiths, 1988, p. 68).

The implementation period refers to the inauguration of the system outlined in the Community Care Bill and fully discussed by Ayer (1990), who points out that research studies (e.g. Booth, 1985; Willcocks, 1987) have indicated that there is a need for a radical overhaul of training for work in residential care.

In recent years various Universities, Polytechnics and Colleges of Higher Education have developed courses at different levels leading to the award of postgraduate Masters degrees, Certificates and Diplomas in social gerontology. Reference to a number of these courses is provided by Ayer in the above-mentioned paper, and the Centre for Policy on Ageing (CPA) publishes a

Bulletin every two months (*New Literature on Old Age*) that has a section devoted to the numerous training courses that are available, and to forthcoming conferences. Readers are referred to the CPA annual list of publications for a very full account of the available literature.

## GENERAL PRINCIPLES IN TRAINING PROFESSIONAL WORKERS

Issues relating to older people in the professional training of four types of health-care workers have been discussed, and it is now time to consider some general principles. These principles will apply, of course, to the training of ancillary staff who take less responsibility in caring for the elderly.

The traditional role of the doctor or other professional has been that of first diagnosing a disordered condition and then, with the individual's consent, initiating an appropriate course of treatment. However, in dealing with the emotional problems of elderly people the diagnostic role should not be confused with that of a counsellor. To take a concrete example, if the client complains of being miserably sexually frustrated, we can make some realistic proposals, but they must be rather tentative, and we must accept that they may not be valid for the person concerned if they go against personal standards and prejudices that are deeply ingrained. All that can be done is to assure the client that there is no evidence that a particular line of recommended action is either unusual or harmful, socially or medically, and to observe that whether it is 'sinful' or 'unseemly' is a matter of opinion.

The professional should be trained to focus upon whatever strengths the individual has and try to enlist them in proposing a course of action most likely to ameliorate the unhappy condition. It should not be assumed that because people are old they are incapable of further moral, and indeed, intellectual growth. Much of the geriatrics and gerontology of the past has been shown by later research to be less reliable than was supposed. Older people can still learn, and the opportunity to acquire new information and to continue their personal growth should be provided by professional workers in their role of educators.

107

However, in training and in practice it must be realized that professionals are not, and never will be, a fount of received wisdom. What they believe to be best for the client, and the policies they try to implement, depend very much on their own personal outlook and philosophy, which is not always rationally based. Their attitudes to such matters as the sexuality of the old, and the propriety of adopting life-styles of which they would disapprove for members of their own family, need to be scrutinized, and one of the objects of training courses is to further such self-scrutiny.

In dealing with elderly people we have the following unique situation. Not only do we see ourselves confronted with special problems in the future when we ourselves grow old, but younger professionals may project themselves forward into middle-age when their own parents will be elderly, and perhaps creating problems in the family. What if a woman in her seventies asks for cosmetic surgery and hormone replacement therapy in order that she can enjoy life with a 'toy-boy'? The young professional may foresee his or her own mother in such a situation in the future, and personally disapprove of it – but how far are we entitled to impose our own personal values on other people in the course of our professional work? For instance, it is generally accepted that young women in their twenties are entitled to some free cosmetic surgery on the NHS if they have unsightly warts on their face, but do we acknowledge that women in their eighties have an equal right to such free treatment?

In theory, we all agree that older people have a right to be treated with the courtesy and respect due to all recipients of professional services, but ageist traditions in the various professions die hard. Well within living memory before the beginning of the NHS, the great bulk of those attending hospitals were literally in receipt of 'charity', with a hospital almoner assessing their ability to pay a little towards their treatment. It is difficult for some professionals not to see older people as part of this charity-receiving populace of the past, and to reflect that they would not have received such 'generous' treatment in their younger days. We may have a long way to go before ageist and class-biased attitudes are eliminated from the professions. Norman (1987) in her *Aspects of Ageism* refers to some pretty extreme examples of the indignities inflicted on elderly people by professional workers in contemporary practice. We need to examine just how far professional training schemes are seeking to examine and perhaps to modify existing attitudes.

This book has insisted that, for most people (although not for all) their sexual life, understood in its broadest sense, is a very important aspect of their total emotional adjustment when they are old, just as when they were young. In fact, for some people the need for love and physical closeness increases in the later years when they are no longer so absorbed with careers, child-rearing, sport, and other activities of younger adults. Many people pay lip-service to this idea, but take the viewpoint that it has already been over-stressed in professional literature (Griggs, 1978; McCarthy, 1979). This conservative viewpoint must be carefully examined, but it could serve to bolster our prejudices against further liberalization of policies concerning care for the elderly, particularly when it is a matter of allocating scarce resources so that privacy is ensured in residential accommodation. Damrosch (1984) has reviewed various studies concerning the attitudes of students and young adults to the sexuality of elderly people, and reports that many of them show that younger people in general are far more tolerant, at least in theory, than has been indicated in the professional literature of less recent times. This might indicate that prejudice is more prevalent and more deeply rooted in more mature professionals, as was suggested in the research of Glass *et al.* (1986) mentioned earlier. As it is the more mature professionals who are responsible for the training of students and newer recruits to their professions, this indicates that continued debate is called for.

## REFERENCES

Arentewicz, G. and Schmidt, G. (eds) (1983) *The Treatment of Sexual Disorders*, Basic Books, New York.

Ayer, S.J. (1990) Who will train the care givers? *Baseline*, 44, 20–27.

Biggs, S. (1989) *Confronting Ageing: A Group Manual for Helping Professionals*, Central Council for Education and Training in Social Work, London.

Booth, T. (1985) *Home Truths: Old People's Homes and the Outcome of Care*, Gower Publishing Co., Aldershot.

Brearly, C.P. (1975) *Social Work, Ageing and Society*, Routledge & Kegan Paul, London.

British Medical Association (1976) *Board of Science and Education*

*Report of the Working Party on Services for the Elderly*, BMA, London.

British Medical Association (1985) *Medicine in Old Age*, BMA, London.

Brody, J.A. (1988) Changing health needs of the ageing population, in Evered, D. and Whelan, J. (eds) *Research and the Ageing Population*, J. Wiley & Sons, Chichester.

Busse, E.W. (1985) Normal aging: The Duke Longitudinal Studies, in Bergener, M., Ermine, M. and Stanalin, H.B. (eds) *Thresholds of Aging*, pp. 215–229, Academic Press, London.

Butler, R.N. and Lewis, M.I. (1988) *Love and Sex After 60*, Harper & Row, New York.

C.C. (1990) Around the training courses: Plymouth, *PSIGE Newsletter* No. 34, 17–19.

Central Council for Education and Training in Social Work (1989) *Requirements and Regulations for the Diploma in Social Work (Paper 30)*, CCETSW Publications, London.

Comfort, A. (1989) *A Good Age*, 2nd edn, Pan Books., London.

Coni, N., Davison, W. and Webster, S. (1984) *Ageing: The Facts*, Oxford University Press, Oxford.

Damrosch, S.P. (1984) Graduate nursing students' attitudes toward sexually active older persons, *The Gerontologist*, 24, 299–302.

Damrosch, S. and Fishman, J. (1985) Medical students' attitudes toward sexually active older persons, *J. Am. Geriat. Soc.*, 33, 852–855.

Davidson, M.A. (1953) Current trends in clinical psychology, in Mace, C.H. and Vernon, P.E. (eds) *Current Trends in British Psychology*, Methuen, London.

Davies, M. (1987) Training in human sexuality in the undergraduate medical curriculum in the U.K. and Eire, *Sexual and Marital Therapy* 2, 83–89.

Deeg, D.H. (1989) *Experiences from Longitudinal Studies of Aging Conceptualization, Organization and Output*, Netherlands Institute of Gerontology, Nijmegen.

De Monchaux, C. and Kier, G.M. (1961) British Psychology 1945–1947, *Acta Psychologica*, 18, 120–180.

Diseker, R.A. and Michielutte, R. (1981) An analysis of empathy in medical students before and following clinical experience, *J. Med. Ed.*, 56, 1004–1010.

Eastman, M. (1984) *Old Age Abuse*, Age Concern, London.

Eastman, M. (1987) A new look at old love, *Health and Soc. Services J.*, 13th October.

Evered, D. and Whelan, J. (eds) (1988) *Research and the Ageing Population*, J. Wiley & Sons, Chichester.

Eysenck, H.J. (1958) Learning theory and behaviour therapy. Paper delivered to the meeting of the Royal Medico-psychological Association, 3rd July.

Gibson, H.B. (1990) Do doctors take the sexuality of older people seriously? Paper delivered to the British Society of Gerontology, 22nd September.

Gillan, P. and Gillan, R. (1976) *Sex Therapy Today*, Open Books, London.

Glass, J.C., Mustian, R.D. and Carter, R.L. (1986) Knowledge and attitudes of health-care providers towards sexuality in the institutionalized elderly, *Educ. Gerontol.*, 12, 465–475.

Griggs, W. (1978) Sex and the elderly, *Am. J. Nursing.* 78, 1352–1354.

Griffiths, E. (1988) No sex please, we're over 60, *Nursing Times*, 84, 34–35.

Griffiths Report (1988) *Community Care: Agenda for Action*, HMSO, London.

Harding, K. (1990) How the system loses good people working in the care of the elderly, *PSIGE Newsletter*, Issue 33, 8–10.

Hawton, K.E. (1979) The human sexuality course for Oxford medical students, *Med. Educ.*, 13, 428–431.

Katzin, L. (1990) Chronic illness and sexuality, *Am. J. Nursing*, January, 56–59.

Kellett, J. (1989) Sex and the elderly, *Br. med. J.*, 299, 934.

Kramer, D., Ber, R. and Moore, M. (1989) Increasing empathy among medical students, *Med. Ed.*, 23, 168–173.

Lamberti, J.W. and Chapel, J.L. (1977), Development and evaluation of a sex education program for medical students, *J. med Educ.*, 5, 582–586.

Liddell, A. (ed.) (1983) *The Practice of Clinical Psychology in Great Britain*, J. Wiley & Sons, Chichester.

McCarthy, P. (1979) Geriatric sexuality: capacity, interest and opportunity, *J. Geront. Nursing*, 5, 20–24.

McCartney, J.R., Iseman, H., Rogers, D. and Cohen, N. (1987) Sexuality and the institutionalized elderly, *J. Am. geriat. Soc.*, 35, 331–333.

McContha, J.T. and Stevenson, R.T. (1982) *The Relationship Between Knowledge of Aging and Attitudes Towards Sexual Expression in the Elderly. A Study of Nursing Home Aides.* Paper presented at the Annual General Meeting of the Mid-Southeast Educational Research Association, New Orleans.

McKenzie, N. (1988) Account of a talk on 'Sexuality in Later Life' by Dr Mary Davies. Unpublished MS.

Masters, W.H. and Johnson, V.E. (1966) *Human Sexual Response*, Little, Brown & Co, Boston.

Masters, W.H. and Johnson, V.E. (1970) *Human Sexual Inadequacy*, J. & A. Churchill, London.

Mossey, J.M. and Shapiro, E. (1982) Self-rated health: a predictor of mortality among the elderly, *Am. J. Pub. Health*, 72, 800–808.

Norman, A. (1987) *Aspects of Ageism*. Centre for Policy on Ageing, London.

Simpson, J.M. (1984) Assessing attitudes towards old people, in Bromley, D.B. (ed.) *Gerontology: Social and Behavioural Perspectives*, pp. 206–212, Croom Helm, London.

Skinner, B.F. and Lindsley, O.R. (1953) *Studies in Behavior Therapy*

*Status Report I*, Washington: Naval Research Contract N5 ori-7662.

Skinner, R. (1988) Young at heart, *Community Care*, 11th Feb. 24–25.

Smith, C.W. and Wattis, J.R. (1989) Medical students' attitudes to old people and career preference: the case of Nottingham Medical School. *Med. Educ.*, 23, 81–85.

Smith, R.G. and Williams, B.O. (1983) A survey of undergraduate teaching of geriatric medicine in the British medical schools, *Age and Ageing*, 12 (Suppl.) 2–6.

Smith, R.G. and Williams, B.O. (1988) Undergraduate teaching of geriatric medicine in the United Kingdom: changes in the years 1981–1986, *Med. Educ.*, 22, 498–500.

Stanley, E. (1978) An introduction to sexuality in the medical curriculum, *Med. Educ.*, 12, 441–445.

Stout, R.W. (1985) Teaching gerontology and geriatric medicine, *Age and Ageing*, 14 (Suppl.) 1–36.

Svanborg, A. (1985) The Gothenburg longitudinal study of 70-year-olds. Clinical reference values in the elderly, in Bergener, M., Ermine, M. and Standelin, H.B. (eds), pp. 231–239, Academic Press, London.

Svanborg, A. (1988) The health of the elderly population: results from longitudinal studies with age-cohort comparisons, in Evered, D. and Whelan, J. (eds) *Research and the Ageing Population*, pp. 3–16, J. Wiley & Sons, Chichester.

Trethowan, W.H. (1977) *The Role of Psychologists in the Health Services*, HMSO, London.

Vollmer, S.A. and Wells, K.B. (1988) How comfortable do first year medical students expect to be when taking sexual histories? *Med. Educ.* 22, 418–425.

White, C.B. (1982) Sexual interests, attitudes, knowledge and sexual history in relation to sexual behavior in the institutionalized aged, *Arch. Sex. Behav.*, 11, 11–21.

Willcocks, D. (1987) *Private Lives in Public Places*, Tavistock, London.

World Health Organization (1974) *WHO Planning and Organization of Geriatric Services*, Technical Report Series 548.

World Health Organization (1982) *Teaching Gerontology and Geriatric Medicine*, report on a workshop, Edinburgh 5–7 Apirl, WHO Publication ICP/ADR 045 (2).

Wright, D. (1985) Sex and the elderly, *Nursing Mirror*, 161, 18–19.

# 5

# Problems with families

Before discussing the problems that people sometimes have with their families in later life, it will be helpful to consider the actual practical arrangements the older members of the community have as to where they live in relation to the family. If we consider people over the present age of retirement, they will probably constitute about 18% of the population by the year 2000. Of these, about 4% are currently living in some form of residential accommodation, and therefore are perhaps living not very near to them. It is difficult to get extensive modern figures concerning the older population who have offspring, as to their closeness to those children in terms of domicile. Many authorities maintain that things have not changed much since the large study of Shanas et al. (1968), and indeed this is confirmed by smaller and more recent studies such as Abrams (1978), Falkingham and Gordon (1988) and Warnes (1984). The statistics given by Butler and Lewis (1982) for the USA present a very similar picture. That things have changed so little in this respect over the years despite the greatly increased proportion of older people in the community, is partly due to the fact that elderly people are now very much more healthy and able to look after themselves despite their age. The chief change is that there are now more single-occupier residences, and many more older women living in them.

The study by Shanas and her colleagues concerned 2,500 people over the age of 60 living in the UK, and selected by the method of 'area probability sampling', which meant that every old person in the country had an equal chance of being represented.

Older people living in institutions (3.7% at that time) were excluded from the study. The findings about family networks indicated that of the elderly who had children, 42% lived with them, and another 40% lived within half an hour's travelling time of one of their children. Thus, over 80% were living in fairly close proximity to their families. Two-thirds of the elderly questioned said that they had seen their family within the last 48 hours. Obviously, these figures will vary very widely according to the district, but they give us something to go on, and to correct the widespread myth that in the 20th century families have rejected their old parents, and that a large proportion of them either live isolated lives or in institutions.

Perhaps what is surprising in the Shanas study is the extent to which older people were still contributing to the family economics. About 50% of them gave 'household services' to their families or made some financial contribution. As might be expected, in times of illness many of the grandparent generation depended on their families for help: about 40% of the population studied said this. As people get older and frailer they tend to live nearer, or with their children, but now that older people are living rather longer, four-generation families are not uncommon, and quite a few retired people are looking after their parents. In such a situation, with the rapidly changing social circumstances over the past century, it is not unnatural that there will be areas of conflict between the generations, even though families are generally maintaining more solidarity than is often supposed.

## PROBLEMS IN RELATION TO GRANDCHILDREN

Two different types of situation causing emotional stress for grandparents may develop. On the one hand, grandparents may not be allowed enough contact with their grandchildren, or a converse situation may prevail: the grandparents (particularly the grandmothers) may find themselves morally compelled to take on too much of the burden of looking after young children, to the detriment of any interests of their own.

Manthorpe and Atherton (1985) describe a young couple who had two children, but the wife adamantly refused to let her parents have anything to do with their grandchildren, a refusal that was naturally very emotionally distresssing for the grand-parents. The circumstances that led up to the development of this situation are not related. In such a situation, the grandparents have no legal rights of access to the children, as in the case of separated parents. The law assumes that, provided the parents are living together and rearing the children in a normal family, they are the best judge of whom their children shall see, and no other relatives have any rights that can be enforced. Where parents are divorced or separated, the situation is somewhat different. According to the Domestic Proceedings and Magistrates' Courts Act, 1978, grandparents can apply through magistrates' courts to be granted legal access to grandchildren in such cases, or when a parent has died.

When a marriage has broken up, it is not uncommon for the parent who has custody of the child to re-marry, or take a common law spouse. The new partner then has the problem of establishing a firm relationship with the children, and the father or mother of the absent or divorced spouse may be perceived as a figure threatening to the new relationship. Whitehouse (1985) cites a case of a couple in their sixties who had looked after their eight-year-old grandson for four years, following the death of his mother. When his father re-married, the boy was taken into the new home, and then the step-mother did all she could to sever his relationship with his grandparents who had been his foster-parents.

These unhappy cases are cited to make the point that while both grandchildren and grandparents can be a source of emotional fulfilment to one another when all is going well in the family, nevertheless it is a relationship that is highly vulnerable by its very nature, particularly in a society such as ours with its high rate of divorce, and other factors contributing to instability. Older people should therefore be chary of investing too much of their emotional capital in their relationships with the third generation. They should not aspire to occupy the role of super-numerary mothers and fathers, but to be people in their own right who have something to give the younger generation by their example, and to help to destroy the myth that ageing is to be associated with a lowering of status. They should not let them-selves be seen as begging the favour of being allowed to care for their grandchildren. If they do give help, taking time off from their own affairs, then it is a favour they are granting, and those in both the parental and grandchild generation should acknowledge this.

## The story of the wooden bowl

There is a well-known story concerning 'The Wooden Bowl'. It is about a three-generation household in which the little son asked his father why Grandad had to eat all his meals out of a wooden bowl. His father replied that it was useless to give the old man anything better, as he would certainly drop and break china. Later, the father heard his little son chipping away in the woodshed, and went to see what he was doing; he found him with a big block of wood, beginning to fashion it into a bowl. 'This will be for you one day, Dad', the little boy told him.

It is very bad for the children if they grow up to regard their grandparents, and all in that generation, as poor old things who are sometimes granted the indulgence of being allowed to help in the house, and to sit in the metaphorical chimney-corner and eat out of 'a wooden bowl'. To some extent this early misperception of the role of the grandparent generation has been one of the causes of the ageist attitudes prevalent in modern society.

Where societies exist with a very low standard of living, as in the village societies studied by Merriman (1984) and referred to in Chapter 3, it is understandable that the grandparent generation, and particularly the women, spend their last years looking after children and performing simple tasks around the house, but that does not mean that they suffer a lowering of status thereby. In some sections of Indian society widowhood itself implies a loss of status, but ageing does not. In our society, however, the transition from a figure of some authority to a child-minder *without* primary authority, does.

How common the situation of grandparents being denied access to their grandchildren is, is difficult to estimate. Certainly it is common enough for Manthorpe and Atherton to write the book mentioned above mainly devoted to the subject. In such cases the emotional health of the grandparents may suffer, as they are being denied a legitimate role, and made to feel unwanted and excluded from the mainstream of life now they have raised their own children. The most obvious reason for such a situation arising is that the parents feel, rightly or wrongly, that their methods of rearing their children will be interfered with by the grandparents. Crawford (1981) points out that, 'normally there is a constraint, perhaps the only one, imposed on grandparents by the parental generation; grandparents must not interfere in the upbringing or the discipline of the child' (p. 502).

Cunningham-Burley (1985) studied 18 couples who were first-time grandparents, and over a series of interviews she tried to identify the various 'rules' for good grandparenting, as perceived by these people. The three major rules that emerged were 'not interfering', 'sharing', and 'not spoiling'. The meanings of the first and last of these labelled rules are self-evident. 'Sharing' means that the amount of time and attention given to the grandchildren must be allocated fairly between the two sets of grandparents, and of course, the parents. How far these grandparents were prepared to abide by the rules in practice is another matter of course, but at least they recognized what was considered proper in their community in Scotland.

That there are potential areas of conflict in families in this matter is obvious, for the child-rearing customs of the grandparents' generation may have differed radically from those that their children are employing. The methods of the grandparents may be too strict, as perceived by their children, or far too indulgent in order to win the affection of the grandchildren. Those in the parental generation may reflect bitterly that in the long term it is they who have to cope with the tantrums and unreasonable demands that have been engendered by granny's spoiling, as dicussed by Labarre *et al.* (1960). When grandparents interfere with the upbringing of their grandchildren, it implies that they are over-involved in something that is not their direct responsibility because their emotional lives may be rather barren. This may follow from bereavement or divorce, or from a marriage that has turned stale and unrewarding, the powerful impulses to give love and exercise some benevolent authority having to find some outlet. Again, as discussed in Chapter 3, the occupational role having been abolished by retirement, a new role may be sought by the retired person who, if lacking in other resources, may regress to a role that was meaningful in earlier life, that of caring for children. That such a role, adopted in later life and invested in too deeply with regard to other people's children, can be very vulnerable and potentially frustrating, has already been pointed out.

While some writers have been concerned for the rights of grandparents who are not given sufficient access to their grandchildren, others have drawn attention to the extent to which older people may be exploited by their children, who over-burden them with responsibilities and chores. Young or middle-aged parents may find that the task of rearing a family has become rather tiresome, particularly when they have developed other interests outside the home (a demanding new job, an intriguing new circle of friends, an extra-marital affair) and look for someone on whom they can off-load their parental respon-sibilities. Naturally they turn to those who supported them in the past – their own parents. It is frequently the case that grand-mothers are victimized and exploited in this way more than grandfathers, because the tradition of our society has been that women stay at home, cook, clean and look after the children, while men go out to work and occupy themselves outside the home. Without being consciously unkind, those in the parental generation may reason that those in the grandparent generation will be only too pleased to be taken notice of and given the honour of being unpaid household helps and child-minders. They are retired from work, and therefore by definition they are without occupation, with time on their hands, and how better occupied could they be than by caring for their own flesh and blood, their grandchildren, and releasing their own children from mundane chores so that they can pursue their 'important' careers, their self development, and valuable recreations? This applies particularly to families which have been upwardly mobile socially, the older generation having been far less well-educated than their children, and who have enjoyed fewer opportunities for advance-ment and self-fulfilment in the past. That the grandparent genera-tion in the UK are much less well-educated than their children, has been commented on by a number of writers. Midwinter (1983) states that 'The British elderly are, in formal terms, not only the worst-educated of any age group in the UK, but just about the worst educated older age group in the developed world' (p. 11). As middle-class people can no longer afford servants as a general rule, the tasks that were formerly done by the servant class tend to be allocated to the grandparent generation.

## THE EXPLOITATION OF THE OLDER GENERATION

Neugarten (1978) makes the distinction between the 'young old', people in their late 50s and early 70s, and the 'old old', those over the age of 75. Such a distinction is still meaningful and useful at present, both in terms of general physical fitness and past educational and occupational experience, but it is likely to be less meaningful as time goes on. Many of the present 'old old' will be dead before the end of the century, and it is doubtful whether the present 'young old' will be much like them, either physically or socially as they age. As Comfort (1990) says, 'Science is nearer than most people realize to attempting the slowing of the health deterioration of age so that vigour lasts longer and death comes later' (p. 25). Neugarten goes on to say that at present the 'young old'

expect that when they grow to advanced old age and can no longer manage for themselves their children will come to their aid – not financially, for the government is looked to as the expected source of financial and medical assistance – but emotionally. As a number of studies have shown, these expectations are usually met (Neugarten, 1978, p. 56).

Many of the older generation are therefore in a position of psychological dependency on their children in so far as they look to the future and wonder who will give them social support and take care of their affairs if they become less than competent when they have reached the status of the 'old old'. Spouses and friends die off, so the relative power of the children increases as time goes on.

Quite decent and reasonable people are apt to treat their own parents in a manner quite different from how they treat other adults. When parents come to stay, they may not be entertained as courteously and considerately as other guests. It may depend, to some extent, on how the children were brought up. If Mother always cleaned the house, cooked the meals, and did the evening washing up so the children were free to do their homework or go out with their friends, it seems natural that Mother (now in her 60s) should revert to these duties – as well as getting the grandchildren off to school in the morning so that her daughter can have a well-earned morning rest in bed. (She's so fond of her grandchildren, of course.) And Dad can make himself useful around the house, catching up on all these jobs that Fred is too busy or too incompetent to carry out himself. This may be all right for a very short visit, but eventually both Mum and Dad may reflect that they had rather hoped that they had left all such chores behind years ago when their children had left home. When old parents become too frail to look after themselves on their own, it becomes a point for discussion among the adult children – should they go into a home, or should they be offered a 'wooden bowl' in one of their children's houses? If the parents have money enough to pay for a more comfortable residential home, should they be allowed to do so? This action may be perceived as a tremendous waste of family money that should be saved and divided among their children when they die. The old parents, having had some experience of staying with their children on past occasions, may wonder if it would be wise to accept such an offer of family hospitality. They might be freer and living more comfortable lives in a residential home, even one run by a Local Authority.

## The effects of parents forming new sexual attachments in later life

The picture becomes radically altered, sometimes to the utter dismay of the younger generation, when a parent rendered single in later life by bereavement or divorce re-marries or takes a permanent lover. Most well-adjusted middle-aged people are pleased at the prospect of their parents leading a full and satisfying emotional life, and, if they find a new partner, having someone special to love and care for them. But not all people are well-adjusted, and some middle-aged children are badly disturbed by such a prospect.

There is, of course, the irrational tendency for children, even in middle-age, to cling to the conviction that their parents do not indulge in sexual activity. Many writers have discussed this curious psychological anomaly, and the psychoanalytic writers have made much of it in terms of the continuing power of the Oedipus complex. Shakespeare's *Hamlet* presents the situation of a son being driven into a frenzy by his widowed mother going to the bed of a new husband, and denouncing her sexuality in the famous bed-chamber scene (Act III.iv). Without invoking Freudian concepts, one may see very well that a selfish and spoilt child who has been accustomed all his or her life to taking for granted the special affection of a parent, has something to gain from this parent being rendered single by bereavement or divorce. But if someone comes along to oust the child from being

No. 1 in the parent's affections, jealousy in its more violent forms may be aroused.

The totally irrational belief that parents do not have a sex-life may cover a more practical view that the parents *should not* indulge in sexual activity. Byers (1983) points out a very practical reason for resentment against a parent's remarriage – that a lone parent is easier to manage and exploit; by acquiring a new spouse or lover such a parent will have an ally and protector, and the whole future relationship is altered in terms of power.

As well as the power relationship being altered by re-marriage, there is the obvious fact that the estate of the parent that the children hoped to inherit entirely, may now become divided because of the existence of a new spouse. In addition, there is always the possibility that if a man marries a much younger wife, more children may be born who have equal rights of inheritance, for men retain their fertility to a great age. Apart from the power issue, and the question of inheritance, middle-aged children may object to the sexual activity of their parents on grounds of sheer sexual jealousy quite apart from any hunger for undivided affection, if their own love-lives are unhappy. A middle-aged son who is reluctantly single, or unhappily married, may feel bitterly jealous if his old father (whom he had regarded as 'past it' and fit only for nursing his wooden bowl in the chimney corner and poking the fire) acquires a new sexual partner and is apparently happy. It is well known that the whole topic of sexuality brings out the most unexpected and strong reactions in many frustrated people. A writer to *The Lancet* comments:

> the younger generation, so liberal, so free, so uninhibited by old-fashioned conventions according to themselves, are often rigid, narrow, puritanical, and censorious when it comes to the behaviour of the older citizens ('In England Now', 1986).

It may be difficult for middle-aged children who are living very free lives themselves to justify their disapproval of their parents' sexuality. The most obvious weapon is ridicule, to regard the whole thing as a tremendous joke. Obviously on rational grounds, children who love, or are at least benevolently disposed towards their ageing parents, should grant them the same rights as themselves, but in this situation children may study how best to embarrass their parents by having recourse to the stereotypes about older people which come so readily to mind. The male newcomer who intrudes in the power structure of the family can be characterized as 'a dirty old man', or ironically as a 'toy-boy'; a female newcomer can be characterized as 'mutton dressed as lamb', or as a 'floozy' obviously after the old fool's money. Lobsenz (1974) writes of a recently remarried man of 78 known to him whose daughter greets him every morning with a derisive inquiry 'How did it go last night?' The grandchildren may serve as a very useful means of discouraging the love-life of an older couple. The couple may be told, in effect, 'You know that *we* don't mind if you want to do it, for we are very broad-minded; but the children would be very shocked if they saw you sharing the same bed, so please be discreet.'

The classic situation of a family trying to control the sexual and domestic life of an older relative is portrayed extremely well by Joyce Carey in his novels *Herself Surprised* and *To Be A Pilgrim*. Here the elderly solicitor, Mr Wilshire, employs Sarah Mundy as his housekeeper, and after a while they start going to bed together. They prove so compatible that eventually he plans to marry her, but when his family hear of this they use the threat of having him certified insane and put away by a medically qualified niece (which might have been possible in the period it concerned). They have Sarah arrested and imprisoned, because they find that she has been pilfering and selling some household stuff, because her housekeeping money is inadequate. That such an abuse of medical and legal power is not so feasible today is obvious, but the sad thing is that some people born in the earlier years of this century are often dominated all too easily by the very different social taboos and attitudes of their youth, and can be bullied and bluffed accordingly.

**The effects of bereavement**

For many people the best means of recovery from bereavement in the long term is to find a new partner after the period of mourning is over. How long this period will be, varies widely between individuals. As is well known, bereavement in later life greatly increases the chances of early death of the surviving partner, particularly for men. However, finding a new partner reverses this tendency. Helsing *et al.* (1981) found that widowers who remarried had a mortality rate lower than that of those who did not. Curiously, their research also showed that the re-married widowers had a mortality rate lower than that of married men in a comparison control group. The meaning of this latter finding is ambiguous; it may indicate that the re-marrying widowers were more vigorous people in general, or that renewing sexual activity with a new partner increases longevity.

When one member of a couple knows that he or she is dying, the question of the future may be discussed, and the person dying may advise re-marriage for the survivor. This seems natural in a normally loving couple. Recovery from bereavement, after the period of mourning, is quicker and more complete if the marriage has been a good one and the surviving partner has little to reproach himself or herself with concerning relations with the deceased. Non-recovery from bereavement is a morbid condition, and Lewis (1989) comments that 'Some women simply become professional widows after the loss of a husband, and do not move in any direction whatsoever – in fact, many enshrine the memory of the spouse for the rest of their life' (p. 78). The mechanism of 'enshrinement' means that the deceased person cannot be discussed or referred to rationally, and feelings of guilt create an unreal halo around him.

It is not only widows and widowers who 'enshrine' a deceased figure; children may have this neurotic reaction to the death of a parent, and then if the surviving partner wishes to form a new attachment in later life, they regard this as an act of disloyalty, an affront to the memory of the dead. This may also occur if parents in later life divorce, and Butler and Lewis give the following advice to those confronted with such a situation:

You can then find yourself accused of being selfish, insensitive or disloyal; and if they succeed in making you feel guilty, you may be compelled to sever your new relationship. This is a mistake. The children need to work through their own anger and grief at the death (or divorce) that ended your marriage. They are often bound to the past by a mixture of positive and negative feelings, and it is this ambivalence that must be resolved. Talk to them freely about their feelings, listen to their reactions, and try honestly to answer questions and clarify confusion. Let them know, also, how you have handled your own feelings about their other parent. (Butler and Lewis, 1988, pp. 141–142).

## Counselling in such family disputes

Typically, children who resent their parents forming new attachments later in life are not dominated by any single one of the reactions and motivations that have been discussed above – a wish to exploit, fear for the inheritance, emotional and sexual jealousy, reverence for a deceased parent, loyalty to a divorced parent – a mixture of all may be involved. Professionals providing counselling in such cases should try to get the children to sort out their muddled motivation, and to gain some insight into the situation. This is by no means an easy task, nor should we expect people to be completely honest in many cases. It may be that a son or daughter has no real resentment against a parent's re-marriage, but has a spouse who is determined to manipulate the situation for mercenary or other motives.

Counselling the older people who contemplate re-marriage and forming new sexual attachments is perhaps more straightforward. The general principle should be that they should be fair to themselves and to their new partner. They should be shown that they will do their children and the wider family no good in the long run if they weakly give in over any issue that will make them powerless or impoverished in their later life. Shakespeare's *King Lear* teaches us a lesson that is still true: that all of us are fallible and potentially weak, and given the opportunity, like Goneril and Regan, may abuse power and convince ourselves that an old parent is not really worth much consideration if he or she stands in the way of the advancement of the younger family. Reinharz (1986) points out that while in *King Lear* a father is driven mad by his power-hungry daughters, the converse occurs in *Hamlet*, where a son is driven mad by the sexuality of his mother and step-father. Some of the issues that may arise in the long term if older parents take unwise decisions will be discussed in the following section.

## ELDER ABUSE AS A FACTOR IN FAMILY POLITICS

The term 'elder abuse' came into general usage some years ago and has been sensationalized by the media under the title of 'granny bashing', and is even referred to in the medical press as 'granny battering' (Burston, 1975; Edwards, 1982). The social myth of everyone loving and respecting their silver-haired old granny appears to be rather stronger in the USA than in Britain, for when Steinmetz (1978), an American sociologist, revealed the prevalence of elder abuse, her revelations were met by shock and disbelief in America. There has been considerable research into the phenomenon, both in America and Britain, since then, but a recent editorial in the *British Medical Journal* states that:

Politicians, health-care professionals, and the general public have largely ignored the subject of the abuse of the elderly. Reluctance to intervene in family affairs, and difficulty in knowing how to cope with the problem when it is identified, are two reasons why it has been ignored (British Medical Journal, 1988).

However, the stereotype that is generally held is of some loutish man beating up his poor old mother, and this is very misleading. For one thing, the abuser is generally a woman, and for another, as shown in Eastman's excellent review of the subject (Eastman 1984), it is not a phenomenon mostly confined to poor and uncultured homes, but occurs with equal frequency in the educated homes of the professional classes.

Eastman's definition of elder abuse should be considered carefully: 'the systematic maltreatment, physical, emotional or financial, of an elderly person by a care-giving relative' (p. 23). Thus physical mistreatment is only one possible form of abuse, and not necessarily the worst; the over-wrought housewife is guilty of physical abuse when she slaps her mother because she has, for the third time in one morning, urinated on the settee in the sitting-room, when she could have quite well asked to be taken to the lavatory. Other forms of abuse may be psychological, such as refusing, for days on end, to speak to an elderly, isolated and helpless father who is confined to his room by arthritis, because of an unresolved quarrel. Financial abuse may occur at many levels, such as pilfering from the weekly pension that has to be fetched for a house-bound relative, and pretending there is hardly enough money to buy necessities, or using various forms of emotional blackmail to get a will altered. How frequently elder abuse occurs is impossible to estimate. Where it is a case of physical abuse there are bruises, broken bones, and over-doses of pills to show for it, but where other forms of abuse occur there is little objective record. Social workers, doctors and others who deal with older people, are familiar with the form of depressive paranoia that may afflict some ageing people so that they tell quite fantastic tales of how they are being robbed and otherwise mistreated by their families, so that it is difficult to sort out fact from fiction.

On the face of it, when we read of the various forms of abuse that elderly people have to suffer at the hands of relatives who are 'care-givers', we may first assume that these abusers must be very unusual and cruel people. However, results of the considerable research that has now begun to accumulate show that this is not the case for the great majority of people who come into this category. They are generally very ordinary people who have been trapped into an intolerable situation by the accumulation of various adverse factors. As mentioned above the abuser is generally female, and most often she is the daughter of the person abused. Strangely, as a number of researches have shown, daughters are more prone to abuse their parents than daughters-in-law, although it might be thought that the natural affection of the real daughter would restrain her, but this would be to misunderstand the situation as it generally occurs. It is more often a female and a daughter, for she is the most likely person to whom the lot of looking after a frail, elderly person commonly falls, and when she is driven to her wit's end by a demanding task that may go on 24 hours a day with little respite, affection turns sour, and she finds herself enacting a horrible new role, at once persecutor and persecuted. Eastman (1984) quotes the following extract from a letter from a woman who admits to abusing her grandmother:

> What do you do when you find that the Nana you have known and loved for 33 years is somebody you don't like? When you find that this cherished person is lazy, dirty and completely uncaring for anybody else ...? You are weary of coping with endless demands, endless complaints, and endless feigned illnesses, not to mention endless emotional blackmail (p. 36).

Although 'elder abuse' covers numerous seemingly identical cases, a variety of different circumstances can lead to this phenomenon. Many tragic situations that have led to gross violence when the carer has broken down seem to be 'nobody's fault', particularly when it is a case of a degenerative condition such as Alzheimer's disease where the whole personality of the afflicted is destroyed, yet he or she lives on as though possessed by a malignant demon who has come to plague the household and destroy the personal relationships within the family. But for the purposes of this chapter we are concerned with situations in which the malignancy is the product of social forces that have operated because of socially inherited customs and attitudes which we should seek to change.

## The long-term results of emotional frustration

The question of elder abuse is discussed in some detail in this chapter because much of it is caused by the frustration of love, in its widest sense, and the failure of personal fulfilment in later life. One could quote the many despairing letters that have been published in the literature of elder abuse which all indicate one thing: older relatives who have been given house-room quite willingly when they were in the 'young old' category may live to become quite intolerable burdens to their families in later years. Reading the many accounts of situations of elder abuse, abuse that is degrading for all parties concerned, one is torn between pity for the abused and pity for the abuser. Where there is no actual evidence of organic brain disease the situation often suggests that the older people are acting in a deliberately bizarre manner in order to take some sort of revenge on those who are caring for them. Where the bizarre behaviour is merely psychological it is bad enough:

> I'm sure total self-absorption and the ability to play games ('I'm a poor dear little old lady and no-one's taking care of me', is the one she can create havoc with) are very common. Much of her behaviour is clearly a cry for more attention, but serves only to alienate those round her. I've shouted at her in the middle of . . . 'You can cut out the amateur dramatics!' (cited by Eastman, 1984, p. 36).

But behaviour that effectively disrupts family life and drives carers wild can involve much worse things than a histrionic demand for attention. Disrupting everyone's sleep, suspiciously inconvenient incontinence, feigned illness, claims of persecution, assault and even rape, are all part of the armoury of weapons

127

available to the malignant elder. Those in the caring professions who try to give assistance cannot always be sure what is fact and what is malicious fiction. Terrible things are sometimes done to older people, and perhaps more frequently when the abuser knows that the victim is less likely to be believed because he or she is a little confused. But even self-inflicted bruises are not unknown as a weapon to break down and shame the care-giving family. There are cases in which the family are quite sure that the bizarre and intolerable behaviour are sure signs that a parent or other elderly relative is now quite psychotic and a candidate for admission to a psychiatric hospital, but after an examination the psychiatrist pronounces him or her to be of perfectly sound mind. Somehow the mask of insanity has been put aside for the benefit of the doctor.

When situations of elder abuse come to light we are faced with cases that often concern the 'old old', and there is little record of what has been going on, say, during the past ten years. How is it that an older relative, who was once welcomed into the family home, has become such an intolerable burden that the family secretly, or not so secretly, wish that death would solve the problem, and resort to punitive methods of which they are deeply ashamed?

The following is not an account of any one case, but an amalgam of quite a number of reported cases, although each one had some unique characteristics. A recently bereaved widow in her 60s who is finding life very lonely is glad to accept the invitation to go and live with her married daughter. At first all goes well and she is pleased to take on much of the responsibility for caring for her young grandchildren. The parents are pleased to be relieved of many unwelcome chores, and the grandmother appears to understand and accept the rules for 'good grand-parenting' that were discussed earlier in this chapter. The increased leisure time that the parents now enjoy enables them to develop more interests outside the home. It seems that this widowed woman has now found a fulfilling role in life; she lives once again in her devotion to her grandchildren, and is in fact more emotionally bound up in this role than she was years ago with her own young children, for then she had a husband to love and be loved by, and an active sex-life which she appreciated. Now she has no emotional outlet other than the young children, and of course, her affection for her daughter, who may not now be as close to her as once she was, having a husband and plenty of outside interests.

This widow's devotion to her role in the family may be taken advantage of by the daughter and son-in-law, who pile more and more work and responsibility on the ageing woman, who now finds that she has little time or energy for anything other than looking after the house and children. While the grandchildren are still young, and responsive to her love, she can accept the workload and all goes well. There is no serious conflict over their upbringing. But they soon grow to be teenagers, and then their grandmother's ideas about what is proper behaviour comes in conflict with those of their parents. The grandmother is shocked by the latitude the adolescents are allowed, and feels that she must put her foot down on certain issues. Her daughter reminds her that they are *her* son and daughter and that she is the ultimate authority as to what is proper and permissable. In the rows that ensue, the more distant past is raked over with recriminations over the older woman's alleged narrowness and silly prejudices.

This grandmother now finds herself deprived of authority, and perhaps shunned by the grandchildren on whom she has lavished so much affection and really hard work at a time of life when her strength has been failing. She has now no proper role in the household except as an increasingly inefficient housekeeper, charwoman and cook. She finds that she must give up these functions progressively as she becomes less and less competent with age. Because she has thrown herself so wholeheartedly into her work in her early sixties, and worked extra hard as she has aged to try to demonstrate that she was still active and reliable, she has tended to lose touch with her female friends of younger days. Some of them will be married and still living with their husbands, some widowed or divorced and living in enviable independence in their own homes, and a few have teamed up with a new man, either in re-marriage or in a free sexual relationship. It is the latter aspect of changing times that can be particularly disturbing to the deprived – the discovery that older women can be sexually attractive and can form new love relationships in later life.

This deprived grandmother now reflects bitterly on what she has done. In accepting her daughter's invitation to come and live in the family home, she had expected to become a loved and honoured figure in her old age, her mature wisdom guiding the lives of the young, but now she finds that she has become just a nuisance, put up with out of duty and not love, and with no one prepared to listen to what they regard as her old-fashioned opinions. She sees, and magnifies the injury, how she has been used and exploited, her chances of some happiness and fulfilment thwarted. She might have found another man, as have a few of her contemporaries, and renewed her sex-life. All the young appear to be doing it nowadays – even young teenagers – so why shouldn't she? But now she is a 'withered crone', a figure who is the subject of vulgar humour. And her ungrateful daughter and family have done this to her! She taunts them with waiting for her to die, and revenges herself by crude acts that she would not have believed herself capable of a few years ago.

That many of the anti-social acts of frustrated older people betray a sexual motivation, is well documented. The drug Praxilene used to be advertised in medical journals with the headline, 'Granny's becoming vulgar'; this refers to the way in which some frustrated older women will embarrass their families by resorting to filthy language in the hearing of the neighbours and visitors. Displays of public masturbation that are generally attributed to brain deterioration (Busse and Pfeiffer, 1977; Renshaw, 1985), may also occur as intentionally shocking acts of defiance against a taboo. The deliberate urination on cushions with the plea 'You know I can't help it' may be a combination of the sexual pleasure of 'urolagnia' (Ellis, 1933) with aggressiveness.

### Preparing a rod for their own backs

The general question of the exploitation of older people by their families has been discussed, and it has been described how some cases of strife within the family that may lead to elder abuse may have their origins in the frustration of the sexual and emotional lives of the grandparent generation. Thus, middle-aged people may have only themselves to blame when they end up having to care for an elderly relative who is outrageously difficult to live with, and who drives at least one caring member of the family to lose control and commit shameful acts of violence. They may have hoped eventually to care for a placid, silver-haired old granny, or a placid and amenable old man sitting in the chimney corner for a few years, until they inherited his money, only to find a very different sort of person living in their house. In a sense, they have prepared a rod for their own backs by seeking to gain a mercenary advantage.

In another sense also, they will have prepared a rod for their future chastisement, for they too will be old one day, and in so far as they have contributed to the ageist tradition of exploiting and frustrating the older generation, they will suffer in their later years.

The beehive operates by the immense and continual labour of *neutered* female bees. These 'worker' bees have been neutered by being fed on a vitamin-restricted diet while in the larval state; only those larvae fed on a rich enough diet develop into queens and become fully sexual. Here we have an analogy with the human institution, which only exists in some cultures and at certain periods, of trying to render the older members of the community sex-less by various taboos, partly in order that their work and their economic substance shall be of use to the younger generation. This is at odds with the declared aims of modern civilizations, as embodied in the World Health Organization (1975) statement that 'Every person has a right to . . . sexual relationships for pleasure as well as for procreation'. This contains no qualification about age.

Possibly in the Victorian era there was less family strife, because women and older people accepted their status that was subservient in many respects. But now the system of taboos has begun crumbling in the twentieth century, both women and people in later life are revolting against the traditional restrictions, and we have entered a period of inevitable family conflict.

**Spouse abuse in later life**

Grown-up children are not the only abusers of the older members of families, and the subject of abuse between spouses has come in for some attention more recently. Years of frustration, sexual and otherwise, can build up in later life, so that although held together by poverty and sharing a common dwelling-place, spouses can come to hate the sight of one another, and one of them may resort to violent abuse, particularly if the other becomes enfeebled and dependent. The abused party knows that he or she can seek refuge in a residential home, but partly out of reluctance to move from the home stays on, enduring the abuse. The following case illustrates this point:

> E had been a battered wife and was becoming Parkinsonian. She tried to get out of a chair, and fell, repeatedly. At first her husband helped her up, but gradually his patience was tried. He would nudge her with his foot, and eventually lost his temper and kicked her. Her neighbour witnessed it and cried over the telephone to the Day Hospital that something should be done, but when asked E replied 'Why should I leave, it's my home'. E's son still lived at home but his comment was 'They are both mad, so I let 'em get on with it.' Eventually she arrived with her face as well as her back bruised, frightened, and she then agreed to go into residential care (Tomlin, 1989).

It might be thought that it is usually the man abusing the woman in later life, a continuation of the 'battered wife syndrome' that is found in the younger years of marriage, (Dobash and Dobash, 1981), however, there are some very significant differences. The violence coming from the male is a very well established stereotype, as represented in the novels of Charles Dickens (Grandfather Smallweed constantly abusing his demented wife; Jeremiah Flintwich giving his wife her 'medicine'; Jerry Cruncher the wife-beater), but investigation of spouse abuse in later life has shown some surprising results.

Pillemer and Finkelhor (1988) studied a stratified random sample of the residents of the Boston metropolitan area who were 65 and over, and identified 63 people who were the subjects of 'abuse' by their definition. They divided them into three categories, the victims of 'physical violence' (n = 40), 'chronic verbal aggression' (n = 26), and 'neglect' (n = 7). They established by means of interviews that as far as physical violence was concerned, husband to wife abuse was 17%, but wife to husband abuse was 43%, a most unexpected finding! The idea that wives use their tongues more than their fists in abusing their husbands was not confirmed, for both husbands and wives resorted to chronic verbal aggression to the same extent, 27%.

The authors of this study discuss various possible explanations of their finding that in the later years of life it is the wives who resort to far more physical violence in abusing their spouses. One possible explanation is that as husbands tend to be older than their wives, and become ill and die at a younger age anyway, they are often the more feeble of the pair and fall victim to physical bullying. In the opinion of the authors of this study, this is not a wholly adequate explanation. Another factor that must be taken into consideration is the question of relative frustration. If we accept that elder abuse in any form is largely the product of the accumulation of chronic frustration in the abuser, then we must consider an observation that was commented on in Chapter 1. It was noted that where the sexual component of marriages dies out in later life it is generally due to the fact that it is the man who withdraws from lovemaking, and leaves his wife to endure years of frustration. Where people are temperamentally given to violence, and their domestic squabbles take this form in their younger years, they often make it up in bed. But when the sexual component has vanished from the marriage due to the man's incapacity, it is natural that the frustrated wife, whose sexual needs alter little with age, should feel like taking it out of him physically.

Too much significance should not be given to this study of Pillemer and Finkelhor, for it was different in a number of ways from many earlier studies of elder abuse, but it should serve to alert other investigators to an area of research that will repay further study.

## REFERENCES

Abrams, M. (1978) *Beyond Three-score and Ten*, Age Concern, Mitcham.

British Medical Journal (1988) Editorial: Elder abuse, *Br. Med. J.* 297, 813–814.

Burston, G.R. (1975) Granny battering, *Br.Med J.* Sept. p. 592.

Busse, E.W. and Pfeiffer, E. (1977) *Behavior and Adaptation in Late Life*, Little, Brown & Co, Boston.

Butler, R.N. and Lewis, M.I. (1982) *Aging and Mental Health*, 3rd edn, Mosby, St Louis.

Butler, R.N. and Lewis, M.I. (1988) *Love and Sex After 60*, Harper & Row, New York.

Byers, J.P. (1983) Sexuality and the elderly, *Geriat. Nurs. (New York)*, 4, 293–297.

Comfort, A. (1990) *A Good Age*, Pan Books, London.

Crawford, M. (1987) Not disengaged: Grandparents in literature and reality, *Sociol. Rev.*, 29, 499–519.

Cunningham-Burley, S. (1985) Constructing grandparenthood: anticipating appropriate action, *Sociology*, 19, 421–436.

Dobash, R.E and Dobash, R.P. (1981) *Violence Against Wives*, Free Press, New York.

Eastman, M. (1984) *Old Age Abuse*, Age Concern, Mitcham.

Ellis, H. (1933) *Psychology of Sex*, W. Heinemann, London.

Edwards, S. (1982) Granny battering, *Med. News*, 11th November.

Falkingham, J. and Gordon, C. (1988) *Fifty Years On: The Income and Household Composition of the Elderly in Britain*, Welfare State Programme, London.

Helsing, K.J., Szklo, M. and Comstock, G.W. (1981) Factors associated with mortality after bereavement, *Am. J. Pub. Health*, 71, 802–809.

In England Now (1986) *The Lancet*, January 18th, 147.

Labarre, M.B., Jessner, L. and Ussery, (1960), The significance of grandmothers in the psychopathology of children, *Am. J. Orthopsychiat.*, 30, 175–185.

Lewis, M. (1989) Sexual problems in the elderly II: Men's vs women's. A panel discussion, *Geriatrics*, 44. 75–86.

Lobsenz, N.M. (1974) Sex and the senior citizen, *The New York Times Magazine*, Jan. 20th.

Manthorpe, J. and Atherton, C. (1985) *Grandparents' Rights*, Age Concern, Mitcham.

Merriman, A. (1984) Social customs affecting the role of elderly women in Indian society in 1982, in Bromley, D.B. (ed.) *Gerontology Social and Behavioural Perspectives*, pp. 151–162. Croom Helm, London.

Midwinter, E. (1983) *Ten Million People*, Centre for Policy on Ageing, London.

Neugarten, B. (1978) Social implications of aging, in Reich, W.T. (ed.) *Encyclopedia of Bioethics*, pp. 54–8, The Free Press, New York.

Pillemer, K. and Finkelhor, D. (1988), The prevalence of elder abuse: a random sample survey, *The Gerontologist*, 28, 51–57.

Reinharz, S. (1986), Loving and hating one's elders: twin themes in legend and literature, in Pillemer, K.A. and Wolf, R.S. (eds) *Elder Abuse: Conflict in the Family*, Auburn House Pub. Co. Dover, Mass.

Renshaw, D, (1985) Sex, age and values, *J. Am. geriat Soc.*, 33, 635–643.

Shanas, E., Townsend, P., Wedderburn, D., Friss, H., Milhoj, P. and Stehover, J. (1968), *Old People in Three Industrial Societies*, Routledge & Kegan Paul, London.

Steinmetz, S.K. (1978) The politics of aging: battered parents, *Society* July/August, 54–55.

Tomlin, E. (1989) *Abuse of Elderly People*, British Geriatrics Society, London.

Warnes, A.M. (1984) *Residential Proximity, Intergenerational Relations and Support for the Elderly*, King's College Department of Geography, London.

Whitehouse, A. (1985) Changing relationships, in Greengross, S. (ed.) *Ageing: An Adventure in Living*, pp. 19–31, Souvenir Press, London.

World Health Organization (1975) *Education and Treatment in Human Sexuality: The Training of Health Professionals. Technical Report No. 572*, WHO, Geneva.

# 6

# Some emotional problems with a sexual basis in later life

This chapter will first examine the emotional and sexual problems that commonly arise when people reach their early sixties, and continue in the later years. Such problems are partly due to the physical changes that result from the process of ageing, the deleterious effects of which are greatly exacerbated by the negative stereotypes about 'the old' that exist in our culture. They are also related to the effects of retirement from work, an important question that will be discussed first. When the various problems have been described and discussed, under different headings, we shall consider what steps professional health-care workers can take in dealing with them.

**PROBLEMS OF RETIREMENT**

When people retire, if they are living as man and wife, the amount of time that they spend together greatly increases, although it may not be as great as one of the partners desires. This change in the life-style of one or both partners can have profound and far-reaching effects, and adjustments have to be made comparable to those which are necessary following marriage or early cohabitation. But when young people adjust to a new way of living, they are generally flexible in their attitudes and adapt relatively easily to a new way of living. Whether or not they have been having sexual relations during the period of courtship, as is relatively common nowadays, the sharing of a home makes some demands on their willingness to compromise with one another's habits, but the emotional stresses involved do not ordinarily impinge much upon their sexual relations. At the age of retirement the situation is very different. Older people may be well adapted to sharing a home, but the home may mean something rather different to the two of them. The man may regard it as a comfortable background to his 'real' work, that is, his paid occupation, and such part-time activities as home decorating, gardening, and other hobbies are generally simple relaxations which are pleasant, but for which there is never enough time. The female partner may have comparable leisure-time pursuits which form a background to her more routine and demanding work whether or not she is gainfully employed. She may have come to regard some areas or aspects of the family home as exclusively 'her' domain, and the man may have assumed that others are exclusively 'his' property. Retirement sometimes results in 'trespasses' in the other's domain, a new source of friction. Both partners may have settled into some sort of stable routine in relation to their work, their homes, and their relations with each other.

Assuming that they have continued to engage in lovemaking, and very large-scale surveys such as that of Starr and Weiner (1981) and Edward Brecher (1984) make it clear that this is the norm for people in their sixties and many older, their sex-lives too will have settled into some stable routine. Butler and Lewis (1988) remark that 'Sexual boredom is very common among older married couples, who tend to fall into routine patterns in which they do the same old thing sexually, time after time, year after year'. This may be so, but most people's work and leisure habits follow some sort of routine, and while they may not provide much excitement, such patterns of habits are generally quite comfortable and peaceful as long as the existing routine is preserved. Upsets may occur with retirement because the whole routine is changed.

It is generally believed that men look forward eagerly to retirement to engage more fully in various activities and projects they have never had time for, only to be disappointed when they find that they never get down to doing what they intended to do, and have time on their hands. The reality is somewhat more complex than this, and often relates to the dynamics of their marriage and to issues that will be discussed later. Rollins and Feldman (1970), who studied 50 couples over the retirement period, found that the pre-retirement period that was especially stressful for men. They write, 'The most devastating period of marriage for males appears to be when they are anticipating retirement.' Once that hurdle had been crossed, after a stormy period of re-adjustment, they eventually settled down to more satisfactory married life. An early study by Burr (1970) also indicated that it was the period immediately prior to retirement that was especially stressful. Much the same situation was found in a much larger survey, that of Edward Brecher (1984), which covered in all 4,246 men and women aged 50 to 93. In Brecher's study people were asked both pre- and post-retirement whether they regarded retirement with positive, negative or mixed feelings, and he reports 'We found that retirement is for many husbands and wives a mere bugaboo – distressing in anticipation but enjoyable after it occurs.' However, of the 803 husbands who had retired, 21% said they had mixed or negative feelings about it, and among the 386 retired wives 25% were less than happy about it. It is the minority that we must consider, for it is they who present to health care professionals with their problems.

## Adjustment of male/female roles following retirement

Even if couples have quite enjoyed one another's company in the limited hours of leisure in the working day, and on the holidays they have taken together, the new situation of being something like twenty-four hours a day together, in some cases, may place a new and intolerable strain on their emotional relationship. A new life is beginning, the life of the 'Third Age', and they are apt to look at and re-assess both each other and themselves. In the past, marital and sexual counsellors were familiar with clients consulting them at five critical periods of marriage: (i) the immediate post-honeymoon period; (ii) after the wife had got her first job outside the home; (iii) following the birth or the first baby; (iv) when the last child left home; (v) post-retirement. The first two of these are less common nowadays due to the prevalence of pre-marital sex, and greater female employment, but the fifth, the retirement period, is now of ever-increasing importance as the population structure shifts with ageing and the number of people retiring increases.

## New sexual conflicts

After retirement, couples who have led a fairly stable and regular sex-life and never bothered to think much about it, now find, perhaps to their own puzzlement and surprise, that sexual conflicts arise just as, perhaps, they occurred in the very early period when they first began to have sex relations. The man's declining potency, the woman's post-menopausal problems (which often have a more psychological than a physiological basis), and the changing physical appearance of them both, provide a fertile ground for such conflicts, but it is the difficulty of role re-adjustment after retirement that is often the real energizer of these sexual difficulties, and fuels the bitterness of the conflicts.

Sexual problems arising out of role re-adjustment are often greater for the working-class than for the middle-class. Sex roles in the former were much more rigidly defined 40 years ago when these couples were young and formed the basis of their marriage. The masculinity of the older working-class man is frequently defined very much by his work-role, and when he loses this on retirement he is apt to feel emasculated. It is especially difficult for newly retired working-class men who still have younger wives going out to work and supplementing the meagre family income. Troll (1971) points out that many older working-class men feel a sense of humiliation when they find that they are expected to do housework and many tasks that they have regarded as 'women's work'. In what way can they now assert their masculinity? In masculine sports? But they have lost their former physical vigour. In bed? But their potency has declined and they may blame sexual failures on the decreased attractiveness of their wives.

Although nowadays there is probably little difference between the sexual practices of the working-class and middle-class as far as young people are concerned, the sort of sexual techniques that are described by Alex Comfort (1987; 1988) were almost unknown to working class people 40 years ago when these older couples formed their sexual unions, and indeed many men would have been quite shocked if their wives had behaved in bed 'like whores'. Middle-class couples are less constrained by the conventions of sex-role division and hence they do not suffer on retirement from the same degree of stress. Also, although attitudes to sexual practices are conditioned by numerous complex factors of upbringing, the 'sexual revolution' affected the middle-class earlier.

## Other problems following retirement

Men may be specially vulnerable in one respect. For reasons that are more historical than rational, women generally retire five years earlier than men. The man may expect to see a great deal more of his wife when he retires, whether she has had a job or worked in the home. However, long before he has retired, not infrequently women whose children have left home have filled their days with various activities outside the house, and developed circles of friends who have nothing to do with their husband's world. He therefore feels rejected and left out in the marital home; his status as a worker is not replaced by any sort of status as was implied by the outworn concept of 'the head of the household'. If he has retired expecting to have a pleasant time pottering around the house being looked after by his loving wife, he may be shocked to find what appears to be a rather different woman living in the house: one who is very busy with her own concerns, who has a host of day-time friends, and has really no more time to give to him than was customary when he was working. She may be as good in bed as ever, but when resentments spring up between couples, the giving and witholding of sex may be used as a weapon to punish and establish mastery.

It hardly needs saying that the retirement of the man may present special problems for the wife. A man who is out at work for most of the day, with his energies largely absorbed by such work, may be a quite tolerable partner to live with, but when he is around all the time defects in his character that are exacerbated if he fails to achieve a successful retirement may become especially noticeable, and in a sense she may feel that she is now living with a different man. Again, the marital bed may become the battleground in an emotional and sexual sense over issues that were not primarily sexual at all. Years of very minor sexual frustration on both sides may now become the subject of bitter recrimination. People of this age may be astonished to find that they are now in need of sexual counselling and information, something they thought was only necessary for the young. Doctors, clinical psychologists, nurses, social workers and other professional workers in health care have long been accustomed to giving sexual information and counselling to young people, but now with the changing climate of opinion, they are being approached more and more by people in their sixties and older. Such popular booklets as that recently published by Age Concern (Greengross and Greengross, 1989) are encouraging older people to realize that they have as legitimate a right to a satisfying sex life as have young and middle-aged people. Professional people must now ask themselves whether they are sufficiently well-informed to answer all the questions they are now being asked by older people, and to deal with the many problems that were not brought to light so frequently in former times. Not a few of the less sophisticated and well-informed professional workers are still unaware of the great wealth of material about the sex lives of older people that is now available in the professional journals. The question of sex education for older people will be discussed further in Chapter 7.

## WOMEN'S PROBLEMS

### The question of physical appearance

Because of the physical marks of ageing, and the mass-media's standards of what constitutes female attractiveness, women, even more than men, are prone to feel that once their youthful appearance and sparkle have gone, no one will ever again find them attractive. This is demonstratively untrue; what makes people attractive in the later years, in both sexes, depends more on the mature character that is expressed in the face, voice and general personality, than the bloom that gives attractiveness to young people. In the survey of 800 men and women over the age of sixty (Starr and Weiner, 1981), people were asked to 'Describe the ideal lover of your fantasy'. Nearly a third of them did not mention any age in connection with their 'ideal', but where an age was mentioned, the great majority of them described someone not much different in age from themselves. Of the men responding, 32.2% described an ideal woman lover as being over sixty. This is perhaps surprising in view of the fact that all these men had been subject to the usual social expectations that older men would prefer much younger women if they could get them.

In fact, only 1.9% of the men specified an 'ideal' in the age range 20–29 years, and 0.4% specified a teenager!

Throughout this book data are cited that derive from large-scale surveys of older people in which opinion questionnaires were used. The research findings of such surveys are very useful, but we must beware of placing too much confidence in them as indicators of contemporary practices, for expressing an opinion is one thing, and actual behaviour another.

Women with deep-seated negative feelings about sex that are only partly modified by attempts at rational thinking, may have been all right when they were young and good-looking by contemporary standards, and having the constant re-assurance of men being obviously attracted to them. But when her body changes with age, a woman in her sixties or older may look at herself and wonder 'Who would find me attractive – would sex with me be "seemly"?' Regarding herself as unattractive, such a woman may gradually change her whole personality, and, married or single, actually rebuff genuine male advances, including those of her own husband. Later in this chapter the means by which such a false self-perception can be changed, will, of course be discussed.

### Women's fear of being left single in later life

Many of the emotional difficulties of older women relate to the possibility of finding themselves alone and forlorn in their later years. If they are married, they may fear that their husbands will leave them, and that never again will they find a male partner. Such a fear may make some women clinging, jealous and demanding in spite of themselves, and so make the situation that they fear more likely to come about. On the other hand, selfish husbands may abuse their wives' sense of insecurity, reasoning that however badly they behave their spouse will never leave them because she would then be miserably on the shelf for the rest of her life.

The fear of being left on her own is, of course, well grounded, since there are many more unmarried women than unmarried men over the age of sixty, as the statistics in Table 6.1 show.

Table 6.1 relates to the year 1987. The final column of Table 1 shows the actual number of women in England and Wales who

**Table 6.1** Estimated population in England and Wales for the year 1987

| | Total | | Thousands<br>Married | | Unmarried* | | Female<br>Excess[§] |
|---|---|---|---|---|---|---|---|
| Age | Males | Females | Males | Females | Males | Females | |
| 50–54 | 1,334.8 | 1,333.4 | 1,105.0 | 1,071.5 | 229.8 | 261.9 | 42.1 |
| 55–59 | 1,319.1 | 1,360.6 | 1,090.6 | 1,035.8 | 228.5 | 324.8 | 96.3 |
| 60–64 | 1,270.6 | 1,376.3 | 1,041.3 | 942.0 | 229.3 | 434.3 | 205.0 |
| 65–69 | 1,120.6 | 1,328.0 | 905.3 | 775.7 | 215.3 | 552.3 | 337.0 |
| 70–74 | 869.0 | 1,170.9 | 666.0 | 522.5 | 203.0 | 648.4 | 445.0 |
| 75+ | 1,143.2 | 2,240.7 | 82.6 | 496.2 | 1,060.6 | 1,744.5 | 683.9 |

*The status of the 'Unmarried' is single + widowed + divorced.
[§]The figure for 'Excess' is derived by subtracting the figure for unmarried males from that of unmarried females.
Statistics derived from Table 1.1 *Office of Population Studies: Series FM2 No. 14*, HMSO.

were unmarried (always single, plus widowed, plus divorced) and 'surplus' in relation to the number of men eligible for marriage in their own half-decade of age range. It will be seen that this number increases dramatically after the age of 60 and increases in the subsequent age groups, so that for the 75+ age group, of the 2,240.7 thousand women living in the country (Scotland and Northern Ireland have separate statistics), 683.9 thousand – 30.5% – are unmarried and cannot be matched with eligible men in the same age group.

However, the official statistics give us no indication of how many unmarried women have well-established relationships with male lovers with whom they may or may not share a house. Because of the prejudice that still exists against older women having lovers, particularly if the latter are rather younger than themselves, women in this position are apt to be somewhat reticent about their domestic affairs, and hence the public image of older women living singly is less than accurate. The fact that confronts us is that many women *fear* to be left alone in their later years, and only education and counselling will overcome that fear.

The numerical imbalance between the sexes in the later decades of life appears to be even more extreme than it is, for if one goes to any event attended by a lot of senior citizens there is generally an overwhelmingly great number of women and relatively few men, but this is partly due to social factors unconnected with the actual sex-ratio in the population. Older women are much more gregarious than older men, and hence are rather more visible publicly.

The social and biological factors that are responsible for the disparity between the sexes numerically in the later decades of life are likely to be with us for some time to come, but already they are changing, and health care professionals should be aware of these factors and be prepared to look ahead to the future when changes in social policies, in social attitudes, and in medical research and practice are likely to further such changes.

At present, women tend to marry men on average about three years older than themselves, and in the past the gap was greater, so there are more widows than widowers. The official statistics show that for people aged over 75 there are more than *four times* as many widows as widowers living in England and Wales. The expectation of life of women used to be reduced by the perils of maternity, but once obstetric practice was improved, this factor became less powerful. The differences in the occupations of the two sexes have meant that men did more dangerous and unhealthy work, and hence had a lower expectation of life, even though in certain sections of the working community (e.g. where women worked in unhealthy factories and mills) some female occupations lowered life expectancy. The trend in the last half of this century has been for the more life-threatening occupations of men to be controlled and re-organized as machinery replaces man-power, so this is increasing the life-expectancy of working-class males. We do not know the extent to which the lower life expectancy of males is due to biological differences, as discussed by Hazard (1989), or due to the less healthy habits of men. Men used to drink and smoke a great deal more than women and this contributed to some extent to their earlier death. It will be seen that in all these instances modern trends towards equality between the sexes both in occupational role and social habits are narrowing the differential, and we are dealing with a phenomenon that is lessening for future generations.

Thus, while *some* unmarried women over the age of 60 may marry, or form sexual relationships with men, this cannot be possible for a great number. Obviously if we are concerned for the personal happiness of single people in the later decades of life, we have to consider whether they would *like* to remarry or cohabitate. We have no reliable information on this question, but it is probable that a minority of both men and women who are single at this time of life, as at any time of life, simply do not wish to enter a sexual relationship, married or unmarried, and many of them will have no special abnormality.

## Problems of older women associated with divorce

Before discussing the problems that divorce brings to older women, it will be helpful to consider just what percentages of older women are single, widowed, and divorced. Table 6.2 sets out the statistics for the decade 1978–1987 for England and Wales, representing the five year age cohorts 50–54 years to 70+ years. This is convenient for our present purpose in this section, and it will also be useful when discussing other matters later in the book.

It will be noted in Table 6.2 that the divorce rate has gone up dramatically over the decade, especially for younger women. As the natural result of men dying before their wives, the percentage of widows increases with age as we look down the columns, but looking across the columns we note that the percentage of widowhood in any age group has not altered significantly over the decade.

With regard to re-marriage, or the formation of new relationships with men, the attitudes of widows differ somewhat from those of divorcees. As discussed in Chapter 5, some widows 'enshrine' the memory of their deceased husbands, and in badly-adjusted people this condition may become permanent. In his study of widows Parkes (1986) found it impossible to get a realistic account of what their deceased husbands were like because they were so frequently idealized, and this is a general problem in bereavement counselling and social work with widows. Reality may become slowly reinstated in the widow's recollection as the process of mourning proceeds, but many older widows are prevented from considering re-marriage, or forming sexual relationships with men, because of a sense of loyalty to the memory of their husbands. It is generally quite otherwise with divorced women, and particularly older divorced women, the latter often

**Table 6.2** Women single, widowed and divorced for the decade
1978–1987. Percentages in England and Wales

| Age-groups | | 1978 | 1979 | 1980 | 1981 | 1982 | 1983 | 1984 | 1985 | 1986 | 1987 |
|---|---|---|---|---|---|---|---|---|---|---|---|
| 50–54 | Single | 7.0 | 6.9 | 6.7 | 6.5 | 6.3 | 6.1 | 5.9 | 5.6 | 5.4 | 5.2 |
| | Widowed | 7.3 | 7.3 | 7.2 | 7.1 | 6.9 | 6.8 | 6.6 | 6.4 | 6.3 | 6.0 |
| | Divorced | 3.9 | 4.3 | 4.7 | 5.1 | 5.5 | 6.0 | 6.6 | 7.1 | 7.8 | 8.4 |
| 55–59 | Single | 8.8 | 8.6 | 8.2 | 7.9 | 7.6 | 7.4 | 7.3 | 7.2 | 7.1 | 6.9 |
| | Widowed | 12.9 | 12.9 | 12.7 | 12.5 | 12.4 | 12.3 | 12.2 | 11.9 | 11.7 | 11.3 |
| | Divorced | 3.5 | 3.7 | 4.0 | 4.3 | 4.5 | 4.8 | 5.2 | 5.6 | 6.0 | 6.5 |
| 60–64 | Single | 8.8 | 8.6 | 8.2 | 7.9 | 7.6 | 7.4 | 7.3 | 7.2 | 7.1 | 6.9 |
| | Widowed | 21.8 | 21.7 | 21.0 | 20.6 | 20.4 | 20.3 | 29.2 | 20.0 | 19.8 | 19.5 |
| | Divorced | 3.0 | 3.2 | 3.4 | 3.7 | 3.9 | 4.2 | 4.4 | 4.6 | 4.9 | 5.1 |
| 65–69 | Single | 10.3 | 9.9 | 9.5 | 9.2 | 8.9 | 8.7 | 8.5 | 8.0 | 7.7 | 7.5 |
| | Widowed | 32.0 | 32.0 | 31.9 | 31.8 | 31.8 | 31.8 | 31.7 | 30.8 | 30.3 | 29.8 |
| | Divorced | 2.4 | 2.6 | 2.8 | 3.0 | 3.1 | 3.3 | 3.5 | 3.8 | 4.0 | 4.3 |
| 70–74 | Single | 12.4 | 12.0 | 11.6 | 11.1 | 10.7 | 10.2 | 9.8 | 9.4 | 9.1 | 8.8 |
| | Widowed | 44.5 | 44.3 | 44.1 | 44.0 | 43.9 | 43.8 | 43.6 | 43.6 | 43.5 | 43.3 |
| | Divorced | 1.8 | 1.9 | 2.0 | 2.2 | 2.4 | 2.6 | 2.8 | 3.0 | 3.1 | 3.3 |
| 75+ | Single | 14.2 | 14.4 | 13.8 | 13.6 | 13.4 | 13.1 | 12.8 | 12.5 | 12.2 | 11.8 |
| | Widowed | 65.3 | 65.3 | 65.1 | 64.9 | 64.7 | 64.5 | 64.4 | 64.4 | 64.4 | 64.2 |
| | Divorced | 0.8 | 0.9 | 1.0 | 1.2 | 1.2 | 1.3 | 1.5 | 1.6 | 1.7 | 1.8 |

Source: Table 1.1(b) *Office of Population Studies, Series FM No. 14* HMSO.

bearing a grudge against their ex-husband because he has left
them in the lurch at an age when it is less likely that they will
ever be able to find a new man.

Some older women who have been divorced naturally seek the
company and support of others of the same status, and it is not
unnatural that they tend to have quite a strong anti-male bias, as
most of them have had husbands whom they regarded as highly
unsatisfactory. Such friendship networks of older divorced
women serve many useful purposes, providing the much-needed
psychological succour to the newly divorced, and offering support
and friendship to retired women living singly in a world that
is still male-dominated and youth-oriented. While there is no
evidence that formally constituted clubs of older divorced women
have been founded, such friendship networks sometimes take the
form of an unofficial 'club', entry to which depends entirely on a
broken marriage, or a marriage that is disintegrating. Women in
such associations are typically living celibately, and rather out of
touch with men, but of course, this does not apply to all divorced
women in the older age groups. Gebhart (1971) found that 43

per cent of divorced women in the 56–60 year old age group were having sexual relations with men, and this figure is possibly higher today, but we are mainly concerned with divorcees over the age of 60.

Lesley Croft (1982) has studied the build-up of anti-male bias among older women. She depicts a female view of men as being '"egomaniacs", continually seeking to gratify their all-encompassing egos by seeking younger women and sex'. While this is certainly true of quite a number of men, bias against the whole of the male sex can reach unreasonable proportions, and Croft goes on to report:

> Many respondents thought it was just as well that men prefer younger women because mentally, they said, men do not mature as fast as women. Although this is commonly said about adolescent boys and girls, it is surprising that this view is projected to the later years and mentioned so frequently by older women. (Croft, 1982, p. 87).

While, as mentioned above, such 'clubs' of divorced women can provide a very useful service for its members, rendering both practical and moral support, they have their negative side if individual women meet a man whom they find particularly congenial and attractive. If such a woman comes to love a man her natural impulse is to relate to him as she would before she was married, but such behaviour might seem disloyal to her sisters in the 'club' to whom she may feel gratitude and perhaps some affection. Part of the ethos of the 'club' may be that 'men are awful', and here she is, tending to betray her sisters with the enemy. Another aspect of the ethos of the 'club' may be to turn the prejudices of the 'chauvinist' males against them, and proudly claim that they are glad to be old, past it, and contemptuous of sex and all that goes with it. Any of that nonsense, they maintain, would be bizarre at their advanced age. A serious conflict may therefore be engendered in the individual woman who meets a congenial man.

The result of the conflict may be that the individual woman who finds herself in this position refuses to respond to any advances a man may make, even breaking a good friendship with him because she cannot trust herself to resist her physical impulses. Many women over 60 and older may be utterly amazed to find themselves falling in love, with all the powerful physiological responses to the man, feelings that they have not experienced for many years, and drawing on half-remembered folk-lore, believe themselves to be going crazy. As will be discussed later, such a phenomenon is not at all abnormal, and professional health care workers can play their part in enlightening women in this position.

All divorcees' 'clubs' do not express the extreme views about men that Lesley Croft has reported, and some of their members may acknowledge, in theory, that it would be a good thing if some of them were to meet a suitable man and form a love-relationship, and even perhaps consider re-marriage. But, realizing the great numerical disproportion between the sexes in their age group, they acknowledge that such good fortune is virtually impossible for all of them, and improbable for most of them. However, although they may acknowledge this hypothetical event calmly, if one of their number actually does give in to her natural impulses and forms a sexual relationship with a man friend, it is natural that she will precipitate jealousy on the part of some of her friends. They may even congratulate her on forming a friendship with a nice man, and gently tease her, but make it clear that they don't know, and don't want to know, that she is sleeping with him. In this situation, the individual woman who has formed a sexual relationship with a man may feel somewhat guilty, and even furtive in her relations with him. If she spends an evening with other members of the 'club' she may have to pretend that she is going home to her own chaste bed, whereas in reality she is not going home, but to her lover's bed. The situation of furtiveness in relation to sex that may have existed when she was a teenager living in her disapproving parents' home may now be revived. Naturally she may feel herself to be confused and ridiculous now that she is an 'old woman' living independently, and with no parents controlling her.

Eric Berne (1966) has written insightfully in his well-known book *Games People Play* about the dynamics of groups, and how the individual member of a group may be trapped into doing what he or she does not want to do, or into making uneasy compromises, when their impulses and actions go against the group ethos. Berne's book and the general theory of 'game playing' is worth studying in connection with the dilemma of an older divorced woman finding herself in the situation that has been described. If the man proposes marriage, that, of course, is so against the group ethos that she will have to find, and believe in, all sorts of reasons why such a step is unthinkable. There are many sound reasons that may apply for an older divorced woman not wishing to form a new marriage contract in certain circumstances, but concern for the group pressure of the divorcees' club is not one of the best of them

## Women in conflicting roles in the family

Women normally love their children and their grandchildren, and in later life they may find considerable satisfaction in the role of grandmother. However, there is a danger that they may find themselves in an emotionally disturbing conflict of roles if in later life, after some years of widowhood or single living, a new man comes into their life. Hitherto their single state, which might otherwise have been a little lonely and aimless, has been made meaningful by their very useful role of being a grandmother. Not all single women, young or old, feel either lonely or aimless, and some even welcome the single state that follows widowhood or divorce as it provides an opportunity to follow and develop personal interests that was denied to them before. However, many women who have had families can find life rather bleak when left on their own in later life. The role of grandmother generally means acting as babysitter, stand-in for married daughters when they are ill, maker of children's clothes, and the welcome provider of treats for the grandchildren.

In such circumstances her role in the 'mum-and-dad' unit has gone, as has much of her role as a mother to her offspring who are no longer truly dependent. But we all need roles in life to give us some validity, and now her roles as 'grandma' has generally conferred on her status, love and respect, and a limited area of power. When a new man comes into her life he does not reconstitute the 'mum-and-dad' unit; her new role is simply that of 'lover' and in some circumstances it may clash with the perceived role of 'grandma'. A state of role-conflict can be very disturbing.

The question of 'Problems with families' has already been discussed in Chapter 5, but this matter is raised again here in connection with the special problems of older women because it is a potential source of emotional conflict for women to a much greater degree than for men. The role of 'grandpa' is less likely to cause such role conflict if a bereaved or divorced man takes a new wife. There may be other emotional troubles if the children do not like the new wife, or are concerned about the inheritance, as discussed at length in the previous chapter, but these difficulties are less concerned with his conflicting roles.

Much depends on the attitude of the middle-aged children, as discussed by Butler and Lewis (1988, Chap. 9). If they have grown to take it for granted that 'grandma' will always be at hand as long as she lives to act as nursemaid and general dogsbody whenever required, selfish children can make their mother uncomfortable and even ashamed of having an independent life of her own by treating it as a huge joke if she forms a relationship with a new man. For reasons discussed previously, they may be opposed to her actually marrying him, but there is enough latent sexist prejudice current to make it easy to induce guilt and shame in women of the present grandparent generation. So 'grandma' is judged irresponsible if she remarries and immoral if she doesn't; she is in the wrong either way.

Possible solutions to this problem of the conflict of roles that may affect older women are discussed later elsewhere in this book. Here it is merely noted among the various social and emotional disabilities that affect women more than men. In later life ageism and sexism combine cruelly to make life difficult for women, yet strangely, the feminist movement has concentrated almost entirely on the problems of younger women, and seems hardly aware of the difficulties that present in later life.

## MEN'S PROBLEMS

### The fear of losing manhood

A lot of the emotional problems that affect men in later life are the result of the physiological changes that take place in the sexual function, as discussed in Chapter 1, and some men's failure to understand and make allowances for what is happening to them. While a woman's sexual performance alters little during

**Table 6.3** Self-ratings of life-enjoyment related to sexual activity

|  | Sexually Active | Sexually Inactive |
| --- | --- | --- |
| Unmarried women | (N = 337) | (N = 155) |
| Life enjoyment high | 81% | 74% |
| Life enjoyment low | 19 | 26 |
|  | 100% | 100% |
| Unmarried men | (N = 345) | (N = 57) |
| Life enjoyment high | 86% | 65% |
| Life enjoyment low | 14 | 35 |
|  | 100% | 100% |

Reprinted from *Love, Sex and Aging: A Consumers Union Report* by Edward M. Brecher and the Editors of Consumer Reports Books, p. 173. Copyright © 1984 by Consumers Union of the United States, Inc. By permission of Little, Brown and Company.

the whole span of her life (despite the popular mythology), except in relation to fertility, a man's performance steadily declines even from the early twenties, a finding established by Kinsey *et al.* (1948)

An individual's self-image is very much bound up with the sexual role. Stimson *et al.* write:

For the older man, an active sex life appears to be crucial to his feelings of self-worth and his feeling that he is respected by his friends and secure socially. As with the younger man, dissatisfaction with sexual activity is related to depression and feelings of worthlessness. (Stimson *et al.*, 1981)

A woman can still regard herself as 'feminine' even though she has no active sex life, but it is not quite the same for the average man. Far fewer men, even in the later decades of life, live on their own or live celibately, and if we consider *unmarried* people's rating of their own total 'life enjoyment', for men, it is very much more related to the question of whether or not they are sexually active. Again, we must turn to American research to get hard data on really large numbers of men and women, and Table 6.3 is taken from Edward Brecher (1984).

A caveat has already been made about comparing data from the USA with conditions that obtain in the UK, but in this particular matter the comparison seems valid. It will be abserved in Table 6.3 that, for the sample of 894 unmarried older men and women as a whole, high life enjoyment is positively related to sexual activity, but the relationship is stronger for the men. If a heterosexual man has taken a pride in what he regards as his masculinity, then, whether he is married or single, he may become very regretful and perhaps ashamed of his declining sexual powers, and seriously concerned that he may become impotent. He may even believe himself to be impotent without adequate reason, a psychological disability that will be discussed later, or have become impotent for various physiological reasons, and feel that this is a great blow to his masculine image. A woman has not this fear to the same degree, for even when she may enjoy sex less, she can still play her part in intercourse in a passive manner.

### Problems of older homosexual men

Some of the problems discussed in this section apply to some extent to lesbian women also, but it is homosexual men in the older generations who have been through most traumatic experiences during a long period of their lives when their sexual expression was forbidden under the criminal law. They form a special group who are different in many ways from the homosexual men in younger generations. While there is now a fair range of publications dealing with the problems of older lesbian women (e.g. Adelman, 1986; Almrig, 1983, Copper, 1986), there is very little published concerning the problems of older homosexual men.

There are various definitions as to the criteria by which we identify a 'homosexual', and we must heed Kinsey's warning that it is artificial to divide mankind between 'heterosexuals' and 'homosexuals', as he found in his extensive studies that for many men some important component of their sex lives was homosexual. We are concerned here with men whose sex lives have been exclusively directed towards their own sex, and we may accept the estimate given by Kimmel (1978) that 10% of the male population are homosexual. As there are now more than 4 million men in England and Wales aged 60 and over, then there are over 400,000 homosexual men in this age group. Considering those over the age of retirement, we have over 300,000 homosexual pensioners. Thus health-care workers who come in contact with retired male clients who need some sort of social care because they live on their own and may have some disability, can expect to have considerably *more* than one in ten whose problems relate to their homosexual orientation. There will be more because most dependent older men are largely looked after by their younger wives, their children, and other younger relatives and relatives-in-law, all of whom are there because of their past history of marriage and procreation. Most older homosexual men do not have such family support and are therefore more dependent on the services of health care workers.

It is therefore very necessary that professional workers in the health-care services should be fully aware of the special nature of the problems of older homosexual men, because they will be coming in contact with far more than they may have anticipated, although they may not always recognize them as such. Let us first consider the myths about the ageing homosexual, and then consider the reality. Various gerontologists and other researchers have attempted to present a true picture of ageing male homosexuals to counteract the prevailing false stereotype (Berger, 1980; Kelly, 1977).

There is the unkind and largely false stereotype of the 'aged queen', or 'auntie', a man who is presumed to have had many homosexual contacts when he was young and good-looking, but in later life finds it impossible to attract sexual partners and is consequently lonely and miserable. This stereotype is not held only by the 'straight' (heterosexual) majority, but it is believed by many of the younger homosexual generation. It is well expressed by a young homosexual man, as reported by Kantrowitz:

I never knew his name. He lived somewhere on the floor above us, rather anonymously. . . . I only knew a few things about him. He wore too many rings. He liked cats and Mozart. He was gentle mannered and fastidious, and he scared me half to death. That was because he was everything I was afraid I was going to be: an 'auntie'. (Kantrowitz, 1976)

In fact, the majority of older homosexual men are not easily recognized. A few, like the celebrated Quentin Crisp, love to be noticed as such, but most, having lived through a long period of persecution in which they risked many forms of social ostracism and legal disabilities, have learnt to conceal their proclivities, and deliberately cultivate a façade of masculine normality. They are a considerable but unrecognized minority with their own special problems about which we know very little. Raymond Berger carried out a long and detailed study of older homosexual men, and he commented:

> Having completed this study I feel more disturbed than ever about the fact that *almost every* gerontological researcher and commentator has chosen to ignore older folk who happen to be homosexual. Can these researchers believe that homosexuals self-destruct at the age of forty? Or have they simply been unaware of the millions of older people who are homosexual? (Berger, 1980 p. 10).

Unfortunately we have little reliable knowledge about the lives of older homosexual men in our society. Although the younger generations of homosexual men have now largely 'come out', so that it is possible to obtain data about them, most homosexual men over 60, for reasons already given, generally prefer to be rather reticent about themselves. Weinberg's study (1970) of homosexual men indicated that the older members of the research population did have less sociosexual contacts than normal, but it did not support the view that their psychological well-being was lower as a result. Although part of the sexual life-style of some of the homosexual community has involved a greater degree of promiscuity than is usual among heterosexual men, with ageing the sexual drive of men is lowered, and they therefore have less incentive to seek new partners. The result appears to be that older homosexual men form stable relationships. Such pairs may not lead as active a social life as most heterosexual married couples, as there is less likely to be an associated family, and when one of them dies, in contrast to heterosexual men, there is very little prospect of the surviving partner forming a new relationship. Hence the prevalence of older homosexual men living on their own, and needing the services of health care workers when they are temporarily ill or permanently infirm.

## OLDER MEN AND WOMEN IN RESIDENTIAL HOMES AND NURSING HOMES

Although only about 3% of the pensioners in England and Wales live in residential homes, the problems that arise from their adjustment to such a change in their life-style demand proper public concern. In general, this chapter endorses the Code of Practice recommended by the Working Party sponsored by the DHSS and convened by the Centre for Policy on Ageing (1984). McCartney *et al.* (1987) have written about the emotional plight of elderly men and women who are living in various types of institution. They note that sexuality is considered to be among the most disturbing problems in such places, and they have found that staff attitudes often lead to difficulties when they are confronted with the continued sexual interests of the residents and patients. A decade ago Roger Clough (1981), investigating various types of old peoples' homes, referred to the temptation of staff to take the attitude towards the residents that 'they're like children really', and to treat them accordingly, exercising authoritarian and inappropriate control. He noted the inevitable imbalance between the sexes numerically in such homes, women greatly predominating, but observed that living in such accommodation provided for those with few social contacts more opportunities for close contacts with others, especially with others of the opposite sex.

Now that we know a great deal more about the extent to which sexual behaviour, actual or desired, is normal among older people even to an advanced age, we have had to reconsider the traditional attitudes to the sexuality of those living in various types of institutions catering for the elderly. Clough discusses the traditional assumptions that used to be made about 'dirty old men' and 'shameless old maids', that have affected staff attitudes. Of one institution he writes:

> In the residential institution the attitudes of staff are of immense significance. That is not to suggest that in an old age home people *will* want to develop sexual relations with others – simply that they *may*, and that staff should know that this is not abnormal, and face squarely any uncertainties that they may have as to what is acceptable. At The Pines the possibility of such a relationship was discouraged in its early stages (Clough, 1981, p. 134).

Matters have certainly improved in the decade since Clough's investigation, due to the writings on the subject of British and American authorities, both medical and non-medical, such as Baikie (1984), Comfort (1980), McCartney *et al.* (1987), Norman

(1987a), and White (1982). Their campaign for the recognition of the legitimacy of sexual expression among the institutionalized elderly has had an impact on the professional workers administering and working in old people's homes. However, in the past decade there has been a great expansion in the number of people living in private and voluntary institutions, although less so in the homes provided by the local authorities. This expansion has created problems in the recruitment and training of additional staff, many of whom have no formal training and whose backgrounds vary greatly. Obviously, any pre-existent ageist prejudices held by such recruits have to be overcome by education, and enlightened attitudes encouraged by getting them to come to terms with their own uncertainties about sexuality. But given a reasonably enlightened and well-informed staff, some problems remain.

One of the most difficult problems for residents and staff alike stems from the fact that in any group of otherwise healthy elderly people there may be a few men and women who are demented to some degree by reason of such conditions as Alzheimer's disease. According to Norman (1987b), one fifth of all those over the age of 80 years are likely to suffer from some degree of dementia. McCartney et al. (1987) refer to the case of a 79-year-old widower in a home for the elderly who was in the early stages of Alzheimer's disease and became very disinhibited in his behaviour, embarrassing the lady residents by outrageous flirtatiousness and telling dirty stories. Obviously residents have a right to be protected from this sort of behaviour being forced upon them. Also, when sexually disinhibited behaviour takes the form of public masturbation, as it does in some cases (Busse and Pfeiffer, 1977; Renshaw, 1985), many residents will find it grossly offensive and look to the staff to protect them. Similarly, when somewhat disinhibited men and women find one another attractive, their behaviour together in public may cause offence to others. Sensitive and enlightened staff will realize that this sort of behaviour is not always best coped with by authortarian repression. Some of it may be due partly to a lack of adequate privacy, for such behaviour need not take place in public if there are private places provided. About half of those living in residential homes are sharing a bedroom, but as Norman (1984) points out, the provision of privacy in such homes should be a matter of priority. The residents can be instructed that it is not the acts in themselves that are wrong, but their public display is giving offence; if people, even if somewhat demented, are treated as responsible adults, they are more likely to respond and behave reasonably.

Some difficult ethical problems arise in relation to residents who are partly demented. If a male resident makes sexual advances to a lady who is a little demented, the staff, and some other residents, may feel that they have a moral duty to 'protect' her, for they may regard her as a young child who is incapable of knowing what is in her own best interests and incapable of giving 'informed consent' in such matters. If the family come to hear that this lady is the mistress of such a man, they may be horrified and charge the staff with allowing her to become his 'victim'. But if the man treats her with proper consideration and she enjoys the relationship, her general happiness may be increased, even if she is not wholly aware of what is going on, or of the shock she is causing to others. Is she truly his 'victim', or is he her benefactor? Such difficult ethical questions demand the attention of a truly mature staff who base their policies on a proper understanding of the issues involved and a real concern for the welfare of the residents, rather than being governed by traditional prejudices about sex and the expediency of administrative convenience.

Allowing individuals the rights of sexual expression may cause emotional distress to some other residents if they are particularly prudish, or jealous of others getting the love and attention that they are not getting. Such people may express their resentment by complaining 'It's not right at our age – it shouldn't be allowed!' Such situations call for careful handling, and imply that further enlightenment in sexual matters is not only necessary for the staff who run such institutions, but the whole community of residents as well. Even if some of the latter have no interest in, or wish for any sexual expression personally, the question should be a matter of public concern, and people should have the opportunity to learn more, and discuss, if they wish to.

Much of the research literature published in Britain and America over the past decade and earlier, some of which has been referred to in this chapter, shows that far from resenting the opportunity to acquire more responsible information in sexual matters being presented to them, the majority of older people welcome it. The general emotional health of those living in the various types of residential homes for elderly people will be increased by the spread of knowledge, and the increased respect for sexual activity among the old. The quality of life for those living in such homes, and the problems associated with the conduct of them, call for a continued enlightenment of the whole resident communities, and social work with the associated families when difficulties arise. There are encouraging signs that more enlightened attitudes towards the sexuality of the elderly are speading among young professional people (Damrosch, 1985), and such enlightenment among the elderly themselves must be fostered.

The question of staff education is by no means simple. While most recruits have had no formal training, a training in nursing or social work may give people quite a lot of factual knowledge concerning the basics of sexuality, but the question of attitude is another matter. A study by Glass et al. (1986) conducted with nursing-home staff, revealed paradoxically that the more knowledge individuals had about sexuality the more restrictive they were in their attitudes. Factors such as education, religiosity, and the time they had held their current positions were significantly related to their attitudes. Donovan and Wynne-Harley (1986) studied the attitudes staff in residential homes had to their job, and took the views of the residents into account when writing their Report. Research studies such as this should be valuable to all those involved in running residential homes and training staff at different levels. Wynne-Harley (1989) urges that residents should be encouraged to be more vociferous in making constructive criticisms as to how homes should be run.

## THE ROLE OF PROFESSIONAL WORKERS

### The identification of problems

Many of the problems that have been descibed in this chapter exist in the community to an unknown extent and require identification. They come to light in three ways: first, by the individual consulting the GP or other professional worker with a direct complaint about the problem; second, by an individual presenting with a vague complaint that masks the real one because he or she is too shy to refer to a problem that has a sexual basis, perhaps fearing that the professional will consider it improper that they should want a sex-life at an 'advanced' age; third, problems that come to light by professional workers visiting the home and inquiring about various matters of health and wellbeing.

In the third category, the professionals who are most likely to detect such problems are visiting nurses of one sort or another, and social workers. In her recent important article, Luker (1988) describes how both District Nurses and Health Visitors attached to general practices were involved in a study where they interviewed over 1,400 men and women aged over 65 years in a 3.86% stratified random sample of the total older population of Trafford, Manchester. About half this sample had not visited their GP with any problem in the three months before the interview, and in the month preceding, 9.6% of the homes had been visited by District Nurses, and .06% by Health Visitors.

Luker contrasts the involvement of District Nurses with the problems of older people with that of Health Visitors, pointing out that the latter generally do not consider that their professional role properly extends to concerning themselves with older people. Nevertheless, Vetter et al. (1986) inaugerated a scheme extending over two years in which a Health Visitor attached to the general practice visited 296 patients aged over 70 years, and a surprisingly large number of emotional and physical problems came to light among patients who had not consulted their doctors. It is evident that Health Visitors can indeed play an important role in rendering preventive and remedial help for older people. Younger women often get a good deal of sexual counselling when they visit family planning clinics, or consult their doctors about obstetric and gynaecological problems. They consider that at their younger age they are entitled to ask about sexual problems. But women long past the menopause do not have contraceptive problems to act as an excuse for seeking sexual advice. They are often far too shy to ask their doctors about sexual matters, perhaps wondering whether they are supposed to be having a sex-life. A visiting female nurse or social worker is in a much better position to elicit and advise upon the sort of problems that have been discussed in this chapter. If necessary, when a medical problem seems to be involved, the latter can persuade the client to see a doctor, and give reassurance that she will get a sympathetic hearing. In the same way, male social workers can elicit and advise upon the sexual problems of those older men who are too diffident to talk to a woman about them, again, persuading them to consult their doctor if a medical problem seems involved.

## What professional care-givers can do

The responsibility of the different sorts of professional care-givers can be summarized under four headings: to organize practical help, to educate, to advise, and to give moral support. In assisting older people to exercise their right to a satisfying emotional life equally with younger people, the question of their sexuality is relevant to most of them, for reasons that have been discussed earlier in this chapter, and elsewhere in this book. Professional workers do not need to be skilled sexual therapists to give the requisite aid. If they fully understand the nature of the problems they encounter, in the great majority of cases, giving basic information to overcome prevailing myths, advising on a sensible course of action, and above all, giving moral support and approval to those who are confused about the normality and legitimacy of their feelings, may be all that is required to enable their clients to achieve a reasonable solution to their problems.

## REFERENCES

Adelman, M (ed.) (1986) *Long Time Passing: Problems of Older Lesbians*, Alyson Publications, Boston.

Almrig, C. *The Invisible Minority: Aging and Lesbians*, Tower Press, Philadelphia.

Baikie, E. (1984) Sexuality and the elderly, in I. Hanley and J. Hodge (eds) *Psychological Approaches to the Care of the Elderly*, Croom Helm, London.

Berger, R. (1980) *Gay and Gray: The Older Homosexual Man*, University of Illinois Press, Urbana.

Berne, E. (1966) *Games People Play: The Psychology of Human Relationships*, Andre Deutsch, London.

Brecher, E.M. (1984) *Love, Sex, and Aging: A Consumer Union Report*, Little, Brown & Co, Boston.

Burr, W.R. (1970) Satisfaction with various aspects of marriage over the life-cycle: A random middle-class sample, *J. Mar. Fam.* 32, 29–37.

Busse, E.W. and Pfeiffer, E. (1977) *Behavior and Adaptation to late Later Life*, Little, Brown & Co, Boston.

Butler, R.M. and Lewis, M.I. (1988) *Love and Sex After Sixty* (revised edn), Harper & Row, New York.

Centre for Policy on Ageing (1984) *Home Life: A Code of Practice for Residential Care*, Centre for Policy on Ageing, London.

Clough, R. (1981) *Old Age Homes*, Allen & Unwin, London.

Comfort, A. (1980) Sexuality in later life, in J.E. Birren and R.L. Sloane (eds) *Handbook of Mental Health and Aging*, pp. 885–892, Prentice Hall, Englewood Cliffs, N.J.

Comfort, A. (1987) *The Joy of Sex*, Quartet Books, London.

Comfort, A. (1988) *More Joy of Sex*, Quartet Books, London.

Copper, B. (1986) *Ageism in the Lesbian Community*, Crossing Press, New York.

Croft, L.H. (1982) *Sexuality in Later Life*, John Wright, Boston.

Damrosch, S.P. (1984) Graduate nursing students' attitudes toward sexually active older persons, *The Gerontologist* 24, 299–302.

Donovan, T. and Wynne-Harley, D. (1986) *Not a Nine-to-Five Job: Staffing and Management in Private and Voluntary Residential Homes*, Centre for Policy on Ageing, London.

Gebhart, P. (1971) Post-marital coitus among widows and divorcees, in P. Bohannan (ed.) *Divorce and After*, Doubleday, New York.

Glass, J.C., Mustian, R.D. and Carter, L.R. (1986) Knowledge and attitudes of health-care providers toward sexuality in the institutionalized elderly, *Educ. Gerontol.*, 12, 465–475.

Greengross, W. and Greengross, S. (1989) *Living, Loving and Ageing*, Age Concern, Mitcham.

Hazard, W.R. (1989) Why do women live longer than men? Biologic differences that affect longevity, *Postgrad. Med.*, 85, 271–283.

Kantrowitz, A. (1976) Dirty old men: we don't want to be reminded that it's going to happen to us, *Advocate*, June 16, 21–29.

Kelly, J. (1977) The aging male homosexual: myth and reality, *Gerontologist*, 17, 328–332.

Kimmel, D.C. (1978) Adult development and aging: a gay prospective, *J. Soc. Issues*, 34, 113–130.

Kinsey, A.C., Pomeroy, W.B. and Martin, C.D. (1948) *Sexual Behavior in the Human Male*, W.B. Saunders & Co, New York.

Luker, K. (1988) The nurse's role in health promotion and preventive health care of the elderly, in N. Wells and C. Freer (eds) *The Ageing Population: Burden or Challenge?* pp. 155–161, The Macmillan Press, Basingstoke.

McCartney, J.R., Izeman, H., Rogers, D. and Cohen, N. (1987) Sexuality in institutionalized elderly, *J. Am. Ger. Soc*, 35, 331–333.

Norman, A. (1984) *Bricks and Mortals: Design and Life-style in Old People's Homes*, Centre for Policy on Ageing, London.

Norman, A. (1987a) *Aspects of Ageism: A Discussion Paper*, Centre for Policy on Ageing, London.

Norman, A. (1987b) *Severe Dementia: The Provision of Long-stay Care*, Centre for Policy on Ageing, London.

Office of Population Studies (1987) *Series FM2 No. 14 Population*, HMSO, London.

Parkes, C.M. (1986) *Bereavement*, Penguin Books, Harmondsworth.

Renshaw, D. (1985) Sex, age and values, *J. Am. Geriat. Soc.* 33, 635–643.

Rollins, B.C. and Feldman, H. (1970) Marital satisfaction over the family cycle, *J. Marr. Fam.*, 32, 20–27.

Starr, B.D. and Weiner, M.B. (1981) *The Starr-Weiner Report on Sex and Sexuality in the Mature years*, McGraw Hill, New York.

Stimson, A., Wase, J.F. and Stimson, J. (1981) Sexuality and self-esteem among the aged, *Res. Aging*, 3, 228–239.

Troll, L. (1971) The family of later life: a decade review, *J. Marr. Fam.*, 33, 263–290.

Vetter, N.J., Jones, D.A. and Victor, C.R. (1986) A health visitor affects the problems that others do not reach, *The Lancet* 2, 30–32.

Weinberg, M.S., (1970) The male homosexual: age-related variations in social and psychological characteristics, *Soc. Prob.* 17, 527–537.

White, C.B. (1988) Sexual interest, attitude, knowledge and sexual history in relation to sexual behavior in the institutionalized aged, *Archiv. Sex. Behav.*, 11, 283–298.

Wynne-Harley, D. (1989) *Speaking Out: Advocacy and Older People* (in press) Centre for Policy on Ageing, London.

161

# 7

# Sex education for older people

Sex education may be distinguished from sex therapy. The latter applies to various conditions of dysfunction, physical and psychological, and these have been discussed in Chapters 1 and 2. Sex education, on the other hand, is like instruction in any other area of human knowledge, and we all need education of one sort and another as we go through life. Adequate education may prevent various forms of dysfunction from developing, and it naturally forms an important part of many programmes of therapy.

According to Stayton (1978) some people put a positive value on *ignorance* in sexual matters. He observes that 'Many segments of our society value sexual ignorance. There is a proscription against knowledge because it is believed that knowledge increases irresponsible behavior.' Such an argument has been levelled against the giving of sex education to schoolchildren, but it can hardly be applied to the instruction of people over the age of retirement. Rather, knowledge of the true facts of sexuality in later life is likely to acquaint people with the risks they may run in embarking on certain courses of behaviour. For instance, an elderly man who marries a woman very much younger than himself may be unaware that he risks having a wife whom he will soon be unable to satisfy sexually, and in her frustration she may eventually turn a roving eye elsewhere. A happy young mistress may become a discontented and perhaps unfaithful wife. Equally misguidedly, a woman rendered single in her 60s by widowhood or divorce, may reject the sincere advances of men attracted to her because, in her ignorance, she assumes that all women of her 'advanced' age are quite unattractive physically and incapable of satisfying a man sexually.

Some people may think that men and women beginning the

last decades of their lives will inevitably resist the idea that they could profit from sex education, and indeed, they may find the suggestion absurd. However, such information as we have indicates that this is not the case. Most people greatly underestimate the interest that older people show in sexual matters nowadays; it used to be a taboo subject which was very little discussed in decent society except under conditions of strict privacy, but now the taboo has been dissipated, many older people tend to feel that their knowledge of an important aspect of human affairs is all too limited. When Edward Brecher and his colleagues began an inquiry among people in the age range 50-93 years for the American Consumers' Union, they were not sure just what topics they might include in their questionnaires. They asked about people's general problems and interests in later life, their health, income level, degree of religious commitment, friendships, periods of loneliness, attitudes towards retirement, and finally, about their love and sex relationships. Somewhat to their surprise, when people were asked whether they would be willing to complete such questionnaires, more than five thousand men and women requested more than ten thousand questionnaires. When the questionnaires were returned, they found that:

Relatively few of our respondents, it turned out, wanted to write about religion in the later years, or about transportation problems after age 50. What interested them most – and what they wrote about most eloquently and at greatest length – was, quite simply, love and sexuality (Brecher, 1984, p. 11).

Starr reports that when lecturing at 'senior centres' the mere mention of the topic of sexuality produces a spate of questions. He quotes four questions, and comments:

There is nothing remarkable about the questions except the ages of the people asking them: 71, 68, 73, and 67. But where can these people turn for help? In most senior centres that Starr and Weiner visited across the United States, they found that sex had never been discussed openly (Starr, 1985, p. 122).

A recently published booklet of *Age concern* (Greengross and Greengross, 1989) has a lighthearted illustration, a drawing showing the notice board of an old people's home. Residents are being asked to choose among various activities by putting a tick against them, and such activities as knitting, bingo, and

163

pottery have collected a few ticks, but the class of 'Kamasutra' has collected far the largest number of ticks, and a delighted old lady is shown adding hers. Although this is intentionally humorous, it is intended to illustrate the point that it is erroneous to assume that old ladies are exclusively concerned with pastimes such as knitting and bingo; sex may be of very real interest to them.

There are three reasons why sex education is especially needed by people in their later years: (1) People in the oldest age cohorts have lived through a period when it was usual to give children, adolescents, and young married people a great deal of active misinformation about sexual matters in general, and they are therefore understandably confused about what is fact and what is myth. (2) Older people have been, and still are, likely to be the subject of ageist propaganda which misrepresents the nature of sexuality in later life, and they may believe some of the myths. (3) When people are entering a period in which their sexuality is changing they need to be instructed as to what changes to expect and how to adapt to them, so that they can continue to live, or begin to live, sexually satisfying lives according to their own personal temperament and circumstances of life.

## (1) THE CORRECTION OF PAST MISINFORMATION

The widespread misinformation about sexual matters that was disseminated by many members of the medical profession at the turn of the century has been described by Hollender (1970). To some extent doctors were guilty of scaremongering, for they had before them the widespread damage that venereal diseases were doing in the community, and the sad problems occasioned by illegitimacy in the nineteenth century, so they felt justified in giving a very bad image of all sexual activity. However, it is plain that many doctors actually believed the nonsense they preached. Alleged 'experts' such as Krafft Ebing were guilty of passing off wild speculations about sexual matters as established scientific fact, and for some reason they fastened on male masturbation as a particular target for their condemnation. According to Brecher and Sussman (1976), Krafft Ebing, in his book *Psychopathia Sexualis* gave the typical Victorian medical view of sex, viewing 'human sexual behaviour as a collection of loathsome diseases . . .

(which) probably did more to elicit a disgust with sex than any other single volume'. The nonsense that some medical men published was eagerly embraced by a great number of school-masters, clergymen and others who were concerned to frighten children and adolescents from engaging in any sexual practices in the name of 'purity'. Baden-Powell's *Scouting for Boys*, in which he preached so feelingly against masturbation, was still being published in its original form in the 1930s.

### Older men's fears about sex

A fear that haunts many men in the older decades derives from a myth that was propagated in the nineteenth century and received considerable medical backing. It was technically known as the principle of 'entropy', and derived from physics. As mis-applied to human sexuality, the theory held that men had only a limited amount of sexual energy to be expended in their lives, and once they had used it up, young or old, they were finished. Most men have never heard of the technical word, but the concept is still believed by many older men. It was preached to boys in the nineteenth century, and later, in an attempt to stop them masturbating, for as Engelhardt (1974) has shown in his interesting review, physicians used to maintain that all sorts of physical and mental ills were caused by masturbation. Astonishingly, quite a lot of older people still believe this in the late twentieth century. A survey of 100 people aged 60–100 years by Friedman (1979) showed that 61 percent believed that masturbation caused mental illness.

In actual fact, the more sexually active a man has been throughout his life, the more he is likely to retain his potency into old age. Comfort refers to some early research work of Pearl which showed that in sexuality 'early starters are late finishers' (Comfort, 1979, p. 169). He goes on to cite the longitudinal research of Pfeiffer *et al.* (1968) studying 254 older men and women over a period of five years, and concludes from this and other studies, that 'senile asexuality' is a sociogenic rather than a biogenic disorder. Later research findings have led to a partial modification of this view. Whitehead (in Barber *et al.* 1989) cautions against over-stating such a case in the light of the most recent findings.

Palmore (1969) found that continued sexual activity in later life was one of the predictors of longevity, a finding that utterly contradicts the old belief that by 'wasting his seed' a man was shortening his life. As continued sexual activity in the later years of life is correlated with general physical vigour, the evidence is equivocal as to whether such activity actually promotes longevity.

## The legacy of past attitudes to women

Women's perception of themselves in the sexual role relates partly to the fact that those who are now of mature years grew up in a past that was still coloured by the extraordinary attitudes of the late Victorian age. It used to be held that 'nice' women did not enjoy sexual intercourse and participated in it only for the purpose of pleasing their husbands and for the sake of bearing children. This attitude was seriously supported by much orthodox medical opinion, and one marriage manual stated the following:

As a general rule, a modest woman seldom desires any sexual gratification for herself. She submits to her husband, but only to please him; and, but for the desire for maternity, would far rather be relieved from his attentions (Cited by Butler and Lewis, 1988, p. 101).

Perry London describes the Victorian ideal of what a wife should be, and writes:

The Victorian wife was to be sweet-tempered, docile, adoring and utterly subservient to her husband, who was to dominate the relationship in all respects. Neither admitted to any sexual feelings, and the more 'pure' their love, the less lustful it was presumed to be. Wifely modesty required the wearing of copious garments, never exposing the body naked (not to physician, not to husband), never naming body parts or functions, never showing passion in the sex act. By and large the husband reciprocated in modesty and language, and did his 'connubial duty' quickly and silently (London, 1978. p. 1561).

Masturbation, then considered a serious disease, was called 'the secret vice'. Homosexuality was considered an unspeakable perversion. Prostitution was rampant in Victorian England, and London became the pornography capital of the world. Women, in most medical opinion, did not masturbate unless they were quite demented, and did not have sexual passions at all if they were quite well. At best, sex was for procreation only, and the more seldom it was used, even for that, the better.

It may be objected that today's women, even in the oldest age groups, were not alive in the Victorian era, although a few were babies at the turn of the century. However, their mothers were, and received an upbringing coloured by the prevailing prudery. These mothers handed on to their daughters, in some measure, the effects of their own upbringing, and although many older women alive today may be quite liberated consciously in their ideas about sexual behaviour and the proper relations between the sexes, they cannot throw off entirely the effects of their early upbringing at the hands of mothers and relatives who had experienced the Victorian treatment. Sometimes such contemporary victims may give a false impression of their degree of liberation when talking to health-care workers, for talk is one thing and behaviour another. They may rationalize their prejudices against sexual behaviour by, for instance, exaggerating the dangers of contraception for women, without knowing much about it, or reacting to their deep-seated guilt over their own sexual enjoyment by believing it does them actual physical harm. Intuitively they may feel that pleasure has to be paid for by pain, and so the various aches and pains of daily living in the later years may be attributed to sex. It is well recognized that all painful conditions, even with an obvious pathology such as arthritis or vertebral displacement, have at least some psychogenic component, and this component may be magnified by guilt and anxiety over sex in some cases and the pain made worse.

### The effects of early misconceptions

People who are now over the age of retirement may vaguely remember some of what they were told about sex in the earlier part of the century, and reflect that when they were grown up they realized that it was mostly nonsense, and that it did not have too bad an effect on their sex lives as adults, once they had overcome some initial embarrassments. In the healthy vigour of early manhood and womanhood, when the sex-drive was strong, they could afford to forget the bugaboos about sex that frightened them as children, but the unfortunate thing is that such early

167

misinformation was apt to engender in them an attitude of underlying disgust of sexual matters, a tendency to treat it all as a dirty joke, and a reluctance to discuss sex seriously. Couples might get along quite well together in bed for many years while the physiological sex-drive was still strong, but be too embarrassed to discuss sexual matters together. When the sex drive weakens with ageing, they may then find themselves in bed with their familiar spouse, but be quite ignorant of what his or her real sex needs are, and unable to ask, or express themselves frankly. Then they may each realize how really ignorant they are about sexual matters, and reflect that the only sexual instruction they have ever received was very long ago and probably mostly nonsense – and certainly very unpleasant. They may wonder where to turn for advice, both for their own sake, and for the benefit of their partner. In this state of confusion they may give up the whole idea of having a satisfactory love-life, as far as its natural physical expression is concerned, even though they may feel that both their partner and themselves have the potential for continued love-making, although perhaps in a different manner.

The plight of those rendered single in later life is made worse by their ignorance of many elementary facts about sexuality in the later years, as explained in Chapters 1 and 2. A widower may be attracted to women around him, but wonder whether women in their sixties would welcome a sexual advance, or even be capable of sexual intercourse. He may even think that women of this age might be shocked at the very idea, and regard him as some sort of freak! Women in their sixties may take it for granted that with their wrinkles, no man will ever be attracted to them again, and be greatly embarrassed when they fall for a man and have all the strong sexual urges that they have not experienced for many years. Such older people are obviously in need of sex education. In fact, they are in greater need than are teenagers who now get instruction very freely from their older contemporaries and from popular magazines, if not in school. But where are older people to get their sex education?

## (2) SEX EDUCATION AS AN ANTIDOTE TO MODERN AGEIST PROPAGANDA

Many people in the grandparent generation have not only to contend with the effects of all the misinformation about sex that they encountered when they were young, but they need to have the resources to combat all the ageist propaganda that is levelled against them at the present time. In previous chapters, the nature of ageism has been discussed, the prejudice against older people that stems largely from fear of growing old and losing youthful vigour and conventional good looks. It has been discussed how this prejudice is strongly reinforced, in some cases, by a wish to exploit the older members of families by taking advantage of their potential for being useful child-minders and household helps. Again, the economic motive strengthens ageism: some younger people act on the principle that their parents and older relatives must be discouraged from spending the family money, and, above all, from forming new love relationships that might divide the expected inheritance. This matter has been discussed in Chapter 6.

Central to ageist propaganda is the question of sexuality. If older people can be made to accept that they are no longer capable of, or entitled to, a proper sex life, then they cannot claim their full rights as adult citizens. The World Health Organization published the following statement:

> Sexual health is the integration of the somatic, emotional, intellectual and social aspects of sexual being, in ways that are positively enriching and that enhance personality, communication and love. Every person has a right to receive information and to consider accepting sexual relationships for pleasure as well as for procreation (WHO, 1975).

Nothing is said here about age. Only by obtaining a breadth of information about sexuality as it applies in the later decades of life will older people be able to maintain their full rights in an environment that is sometimes hostile to them.

### (3) UNDERSTANDING CHANGES TAKING PLACE IN THEMSELVES AND THEIR PARTNER

Without instruction, men and women enter the last decades of their lives very vulnerable to all sorts of misunderstandings about sex that are likely to lead to unhappiness for both themselves and their partners. If they expect to continue to lead the same sort of sex-life that they had in middle-age they will be sadly disappointed, and if they do not realize the sort of changes that may take place in both men and women, they will become very inadequate lovers. In general, people do not expect to continue to make love as they did in middle age, but they are often very unsure as to what will happen. Some men expect to become impotent after the age of about 50 or 60, and here they may be a prey to some scare advertising that has been appearing in the press very recently. A commercial firm that advertises its services in preserving or restoring potency makes the following misleading statement in its publicity brochure:

> Thanks to a revolutionary breakthrough male impotence can now be successfully treated in nine cases out of ten.
>
> This distressing condition is more common than most people imagine. Ten per cent of all men are affected and up to 40% of those over the age of 50.

This is scare advertising, intended to frighten people into coming for treatment. To claim that 'ten per cent of all men are affected' is virtually meaningless. First, they do not define 'impotence'; failure to achieve or maintain erection on all occasions, or one occasion in ten, or one in 100? Second, to say that 'up to 40% of those over the age of 50', are affected, is rubbish. What does 'up to' mean? The percentage affected depends upon the particular age cohort that is being studied. Finally, it is absurd to make a claim that successful treatment can be given to 'nine cases out of ten'. This would certainly not be true if all their clients were in their 90s! The treatment this clinic offers, according to their publicity brochure, is 'Pharmacologically Induced Penile Erection' which probably means the injection of papaverine or similar agents into the penis, a technique that has been mentioned, along with its dangers, in Chapter 1. As has already been explained, men who do not properly understand what is happening to them in the normal course of ageing may suffer from one or two incidents of failure to achieve erection and fear that they are becoming impotent. Such a fear may very well produce performance anxiety which can cause psychogenic impotence. No doubt advertisers of commercial treatments, such as that mentioned above, hope to attract such cases as clients.

Not only do men need to be instructed as to what physiological changes they may expect to take place in their own bodies, and how to cope with them, but they need to understand what happens to women in order to be effective and considerate lovers. Most men probably underestimate the capacity for enjoyment and sexual performance in older women. They are aware that their own sexual performance is declining, and so expect a comparable decline to take place in women, which is not the case. They may not be aware that if a decline in sexual capacity in women follows the menopause, this can generally be rectified quite easily by hormone replacement therapy.

Women also need to know about men. In their younger years they may have come to regard men as robust and ever-ready studs, who could be expected to do all the wooing to bring on the conventionally reluctant female. In later life the roles may become somewhat reversed in this respect, the sexuality of the woman being the more robust, and that of the man more subject to subtle psychological influences. Sometimes the sex instruction manuals that are written for younger adults make statements that are not entirely true for older people. Thus Williams (1986) states that 'A woman's desire and responsiveness tends to be even more susceptible to psychological influences, internal and external, than a man's. As the saying goes, "Biology moves her but psychology rules her!"' (p. 33). Allowing for the fact that there are enormous individual differences, this male/female contrast is less true in later life, and in many cases the reverse is true, older women being tougher. Williams goes on to admit that:

> We must all understand and accept that getting older produces changes in our pattern of sexual interest and responsiveness, and one crucial change is that we simply have to begin paying attention to our conditions for being interested and responsive. *This becomes progressively more important as we get older* (p. 34).

Sometimes a man may eschew love-making entirely because he feels that he cannot live up to his previous standards of performance. This creates a most unfortunate social situation. If older men fear the 'challenge' of a situation in which their sexual potency will be put to the test, then they may withdraw from socialization with women, as well as from sexual encounters with them, and this exacerbates a problem that already exists – that there are already four times as many *single* women as *single* men after the age of 65, as discussed in the previous chapter. Unless both men and women in the later years of life have adequate knowledge about sexuality, the relations between the two sexes is beset with pitfalls.

## TOWARDS A NEW CONCEPT OF SEXUALITY

When people enter the later decades of life, they should consider what sex means to them. There are many problems associated with the continuance of sexual activity in later life, or its renewal after a period of celibacy following widowhood. It may be questioned whether older people should not resign themselves to living celibate lives in some circumstances; if married, to continue marital relations for the sake of companionship, but not worry if the physical aspect of the marriage comes to a complete end. If they find themselves rendered single, should they aspire to form new sexual relationships? After all, it is admitted that the physiological drive for sex dies down in intensity with age, at least with men, and it may seem that there is little point in stoking, rather than damping down, a furnace that can lead to all sorts of social inconveniences.

It is entirely understandable if some people see the situation in these terms, and as active professional health-care workers are mostly young or middle-aged, they may find it difficult to understand just what is being asked of them in the new thinking that is being pioneered in this and similar books and journals. Is it right, they may ask, if organizations such as Age Concern encourage the grandparent generation to expect to lead a full sex-life, and to demand the attention of professional workers to their alleged needs?

To consider this question, it is necessary to explain a concept of sexuality that applies in later life, and is rather different from that which characterizes the younger years of adulthood. Most older people may take some time fully to realize the physiological and psychosocial changes that will take place over perhaps the last 30 years of their lives, and if they hope to recapture precisely the same sort of sexual satisfactions that they had in youth and middle-age, they will be disappointed. Yet sexuality in later life can be fulfilling and of great importance to many people, although some people at all ages seem to lead well-adjusted asexual lives.

Throughout life most people need to regard themselves positively with regard to their feminine or masculine sexuality. This is generally a deep psychological need, and denial of it may lead to depression and preternatural ageing. As people age, they are subject to subtle psychosocial changes, as well as to physiological changes. If a man tries to cling to a macho image of being a frequent and efficient phallic performer, he is heading for trouble, and may perhaps suffer from performance anxiety, so that eventually he comes to regard himself as impotent, and withdraws from love-making altogether. But with a more sophisticated understanding of the expression of emotional feeling in physical terms, he may enjoy a lifetime of rewarding love-making in which phallic performance, appropriate to his age, need not play such a major part. With a woman, the problem is different, but there is no reason why she should ever lose her sense of femininity, or to cease to be attractive to the right person despite her increasing wrinkles.

To most people, sex means copulation with the goal of the male orgasm, conceived of as the ejaculation of semen. Although most intercourse is engaged in not for procreation but for re-creation, this goal is over-emphasized. However, this traditional view of sex has been becoming modified over the more recent decades, partly due to the feminist movement, but also due to the work of sex researchers and therapists. When sex therapists have asked people what they really want of sex, the answer appears to be pleasure, satisfaction, psychological contentment. These are the real goals of love-making, rather than the limited traditional goal. McCarthy (1977) points out that the language which many people use in referring to sexual activity emphasizes the 'getting to' rather than the 'experiencing of' a pleasurable activity. He points out that the terms 'foreplay' and 'afterplay' emphasize that there is a 'big event' as a goal which has to be reached, and all else is subsidiary. Some feminists have complained angrily of the male definition of sex – that it lasts 'until *he* comes' and then it is all over.

The emphasis on peno-vaginal intercourse culminating in male orgasm as being the essential and defining characteristic of love-making is regarded by many feminists such as Hite (1976) as merely fulfilling a macho male need to boost their masculinity. Her investigations of female sexuality showed that many women's feelings of fulfilment in sex depended on a far broader range of activities involving intimate sexual techniques. There are, in fact, some women who have never experienced orgasm in intercourse, but who have experienced it regularly or occasionally through manual or oral contacts in lovemaking. One of the greatest benefits a counsellor can confer on an ageing man is to get him to realize that his masculinity does not depend wholly on his phallic prowess, and that an experienced lover will be able to give and receive sensual pleasure and emotional satisfaction through the wide range of lovemaking techniques that are generally known by sex therapists as 'pleasuring' (Cooper, 1988; Gochros and Fisher, 1980; Kaplan, 1974; Kass and Strauss, 1975; LoPiccolo, 1978; Starr, 1985; Starr and Weiner, 1981; Sviland, 1978).

It is not suggested here that all health care professionals need to become experts in sex therapy, but merely that they should know enough to discard the old equation expressed thus: 'The equation for men with this view that sex = erection plus intercourse, along with its corollary of no erection = no sex, is perceived as logical and absolute.' (Starr, 1985, p. 115). The new orientation of modern sex therapists that is necessary in advising older people to regard intercourse as desirable, but not an essential component of lovemaking. One such therapist, Grahame Cooper, writes thus:

> Learning to integrate foreplay and intercourse, perhaps for the first time, is an important educative component of the new sex therapies, and it helps to correct the misconception that foreplay is something that the man does to the woman in order to get her ready for him to penetrate her in sexual intercourse. Rather, the aim is to achieve a level of physical and emotional interaction between the couple, enhanced by open communication, which will lead to increased pleasure for both of them in the course of which the woman will become sufficiently sexually aroused for *acceptance* of the penis into her vagina to occur comfortably and pleasurably. For the man it is hoped that the increased pleasure will lead to sufficient erection of the penis for it to be contained and retained within the vagina during the movements of sexual intercourse. This statement does not preclude the possibility that some couples achieve their sexual pleasure without genital intercourse, nor does it exclude the fact that genital intercourse is perfectly feasible with a flaccid penis, provided that the woman is in a

sufficient state of sexual arousal to accept it vaginally. (Cooper, 1988, p. 135).

Older men should ask themselves 'What do I need sex *for* – is it a compulsive effort to demonstrate to myself and others that I am not yet a worn out "old man" '? Many people use the rituals of love-making for purposes that are basically a-sexual. Some researchers such as Denny *et al.* (1984) have found that even among younger people, many women enjoy the total experience involving all sorts of caressing, which is generally known as 'fore-play', as much as, or more than, the act of intercourse. Younger men tend to say that that the act of intercourse is more important to them, but this may reflect a strong psychological as well as a physical need, and it may not apply to older lovers if they are happy about their male identity and feel no need to prove themselves.

When a married man with the totally conventional and limited view of sex (which is now common only among men of the older generations), finds that his phallic performance is declining with age, he may, as discussed earlier, withdraw entirely from all sexual encounters out of pride. His wife may still be as ready for love-making in all its aspects as she ever was, but she may have to endure a total deprivation for many years because of her husband's 'impotence'. This cruel deprivation may be interpreted by her as being all her fault, attributing it to her ageing appearance, and there are many men who will give this as a reason for their withdrawal from sexual relations. Starr (1985) refers to 'the tyranny that the male erection holds over the potential for intimacy, physical stimulation, and sexual pleasuring', and goes on to write:

Pleasuring refers to any sexual experience that feels good. With pleasuring there is no one act that measures or validates the success of the experience. There are just different events, intercourse and orgasm being just two, neither of which is necessary or essential for a pleasurable experience. Within the context of the pleasuring definition of sexuality, adults of all ages are on an equal par. Frequency and degree of sexual pleasure are limited only by interest, desire, and imagination. While the frequency of different acts may vary, (e.g some may have more frequent intercourse than others), the potential for pleasuring is open to couples with whatever frequency is desired, regardless of erectile response or age. From this point of view, some of those who seek and achieve intercourse could conceivably experience less pleasure and, therefore, less sexuality than those open to and skillful at a variety of forms of sexual pleasuring (pp. 115–116).

Full credit must be given to the original studies of Masters and Johnson (1966) who, in their therapy for younger couples, popularized the idea of 'pleasuring' without intercourse as a valuable aspect of love-making that may, or may not, lead to intercourse.

Sex education in later life may therefore come as a great liberating influence in the lives of many men and women, relieving them of guilt and pressure to perform to an unrealistic standard. It is liberating to realize that there are enormous natural variations between people, and between couples, as to their expression of sexuality, as became apparent from the early studies of Kinsey and his colleagues. Older people need liberating from all sorts of irrational taboos: for instance, a woman in her seventies may begin to suffer from arthritis, which makes it painful to spread her legs in the face-to-face position of intercourse that she has enjoyed all her adult life. She may never have copulated in any other position, and indeed, have regarded other positions (if she has heard of them!) as being somewhat 'perverse' and not within the province of decent sexual relations. Her husband may be too shy to urge her to vary their usual practice, regretfully accepting that they must abandon all intercourse because of her arthritis. It needs to be pointed out to such a couple by an authoritative professional person that their difficulty may be solved by using other techniques, such as the man lying behind his partner, and that such a position is neither 'perverse' nor uncommon. Similarly, all sorts of sexual techniques that are described in modern sex instruction books, that younger people practise for fun and for variety, are very suitable for older people whose minor disabilities make the continuance of their usual forms of love-making more difficult. Here we come to one of the great difficulties in imparting knowledge in this important aspect of health-care to many, although not to all, older people. Some may say, in effect, 'But surely such antics are only for the young – it would be unseemly for us to behave in such a way, or even to discuss it together!'

## HOW DO WE IMPART SEX EDUCATION TO OLDER PEOPLE?

The following incident illustrates a very real problem. There is an organization, the University of the Third Age, which now has autonomous branches in quite a number of countries, and caters for the interests and activities of people who are mainly, although not entirely, over the age of retirement. At a recent international conference convened by a branch in a university city, there were various eminent speakers lecturing on topics of special interest to older people. It was announced that many of these speakers had books of their authorship on display and available at a nearby bookshop, and attenders at the conference were invited to go there, browse, and buy them. These books attracted some attention, and there was quite a sale of them, with the exception of one author. This was Alex Comfort, whose talk was much appreciated, but the only two books of his the bookshop displayed were *The Joy of Sex* (1987) and *More Joy of Sex* (1988), which were left severely alone. These two books, although they contain some sensible facts and advice on ageing, are lavishly and quite tastefully illustrated with drawings of young and comely men and women making love in a great variety of ways, and this is enough to put off many older people from buying them openly, or to be seen reading them in a bookshop. A lady in her 60s, known to the present author, has one of them in a brown envelope in her desk, whereas a younger woman might display it openly on her bookshelf, without giving much thought to its presence.

Earlier in this chapter reference was made to a humorous cartoon showing an old lady adding her tick to the many others responding to the offer of classes in the Kamasutra in an old people's home. This represents the wish, rather than the reality, but it would be interesting to see how such an offer would be received if it were really offered among the other interesting activities in such a home.

It is difficult, therefore, to get the older generation to buy, borrow or read books of sex instruction, even though they may be quite educated people. They are embarrassed to be reading such books at their age. In the 1920s and 1930s when such books came widely on the market, they were often sold in 'rubber goods' shops, along with condoms, douches and Dameroids, or sold in back-street bookshops which dealt in surreptitious pornography, and they may still retain this image in the minds of many older people. The fact that Comfort's sex books are now attractively presented and sold openly in respectable bookshops is all to the good, but their bold appeal to the young makes older people shy of reading them. Comfort's re-issued paperback *A Good Age* (1990) (first published in 1977) is well illustrated with pictures of older people, but none of them are making love, and there is a good section on sexuality in ageing. Age Concern have published *Living, Loving and Ageing* (Greengross and Greengross, 1989) which is directed to the reading public and is mainly about the sex lives of older people, offering much sensible advice. One criticism may be made of this book: it unintentionally presents a rather negative image of sexuality in later life because it highlights all the things that can go wrong, failing to indicate just how rare these morbid conditions are. The senior author, Wendy Greengross, is a medical doctor with a reputation for helping the handicapped (Greengross, 1982), so it is natural that her experience of older people will be atypical. Since doctors are primarily concerned with the sick and the handicapped, they have less experience with the healthy old who are the majority and have less need of their services. Their book deals in considerable detail with various conditions such as amputated penises, faecal incontinence, implanted catheters, colostomy, prolapsed vaginas and suchlike, and some readers will find these passages grisly reading.

Obviously the unfortunate people who have such conditions need help and advice regarding their sex-lives, but discussion in a doctor's surgery, or with a visiting health-care professional, would seem to be the appropriate situation, rather than in a popular paperback. Some people who are approaching later life may get the impression from this book that all these disabilities may be in store for them and their partners as they age, and reflect that they would rather give up love-making altogether than have to cope with the handicaps attendant on faecal incontinence, an implanted catheter, a prolapsed vagina etc.! It must be emphasized that the main impediments to a satisfying love life in our later years are not *physical* at all, but *psychological*, the product of the negative image that sex in later life has in most people's perception of it, and that what is chiefly needed is to improve this image.

There is a dearth of good books dealing with sex in later life, and directed to the reading public of average intelligence. A short list is given in Appendix A, but it should be noted that as some are published in America and Australia, it is not easy to get them in the UK. But however good the supply of sex education books suitable for older people is, there is the problem that it is not always easy to get people in the older generation to read them. They would like the information, but are reluctant to get it from a book. Professional health-care givers have therefore to study how and when to give it by word of mouth.

Hawton (1985) makes the point that in providing advice to older couples about sexual matters:

> It is unwise to assume that a couple have a sophisticated knowledge of sexuality; very often a couple who give this impression will be unwilling to admit to areas of ignorance, or be unaware of their blindspots. A fairly didactic educational session, in which pictures are used, is helpful. This session should be tailored to needs and problems, as well as the educational level, of the individual couple (p. 182).

The paradox here is that more educated and superficially sophisticated people may be the ones more prone to pretend to a greater knowledge of sexuality than they possess, whereas less educated and simpler men and women may freely admit to the extent of their ignorance.

One aspect of providing advice and education to people of more limited general education is that their sexual vocabulary may be very different from that of the professional person giving the instruction. While less educated people may not know the meaning of words such as 'vulva' or 'fellatio' – or have an inaccurate knowledge of what they mean – professional people may not know the vernacular terms commonly used by their clients, and which vary from district to district. A further difficulty arises because some vernacular terms serve the double function of referring to sexual organs and practices, and of being coarse swear-words. A working-class man or woman, particularly of the older generation, might be very shocked to hear a professional person using such vernacular terms, and it requires some experience and tact in acquiring a vocabulary of words that are 'acceptable' demotic terms that refer to sexual parts and functions in a particular part of the country. Felstein (1986, Chapter 2) gives an intelligent discussion of this question and provides a glossary of various demotic sexual terms. When health-care professionals have acquired a vocabulary of words that are acceptable in a particular part of the country, they will find that provided such terms are used by them without embarrassment, clients will be grateful to them for being so frank, and they will be able to discuss intimate matters freely.

It is obvious that the question of whether individuals will be better instructed by means of books or by word of mouth must be left to the judgement of the professional. In many cases both are necessary. Books give the facts in black and white, and clients can always come back and ask for anything they do not understand to be explained, but the difficulties of getting people to read books have been discussed. In books clients may come across descriptions of certain sexual practices they have never heard of before and exclaim, 'How dreadful – I could never do that!' whereas when it is carefully explained by a sympathetic person whose authority they respect, then they feel they have 'permission' to engage in the activity in question and see if it suits them. Health-care professionals should, of course, avoid any suggestion of 'evangelism', as is well put by Dr Kellett who writes:

> The sexuality of the elderly is no place for the evangelist. The recognition that continued physical intimacy benefits both the psychological and physical health of the individual must be tempered by a willingness to allow elderly people to make their own decisions unpressured by those who are younger. The embarrassment of the patients will be overcome only if the doctor can take the lead in introducing the topic – which is not easy for those of us who have been taught that elderly people don't do it (Kellett, 1989 p. 934).

It is, of course, up to all individuals to decide how they conduct their own lives, whether they have a sex-life at all, and what form it shall take. All professionals can do, and should do, is to assist them to make informed choices in the light of modern knowledge and the facilities available. It need hardly be stressed that in taking the lead, the professional should then be prepared to *listen* rather than continuing to talk didactically. The skill of getting patients and clients to talk comes with practice, and the professional may continue to learn a lot by listening to elderly people who, although they may lack their education and training, have had a long experience of life.

# REFERENCES

Barber, H.R.K., Butler, R.N., Lewis, M. *et al.* (1989) Sexual problems in the elderly. II Men's vs Women's. *Geriatrics*, 44, 75–86.

Brecher, E.M. (1984) *Love, Sex and Aging: A Consumer Union Report*, Little, Brown & Co, Boston.

Brecher, E.M. and Sussman, N. (1976) History of human sexual research and study, in Sadcock, B.J. and Freedman, A.M. (eds) *The Sexual Experience*, p. 7, Williams & Wilkins, Baltimore.

Butler R.N. and Lewis, M.I. (1988) *Love and Sex After 60*, Harper & Row, New York.

Comfort, A. (1979) *The Biology of Senescence*, Elsevier, New York.

Comfort, A. (1987) *The Joy of Sex*, Quartet Books, London.

Comfort, A. (1988) *More Joy of Sex*, Quartet Books, London.

Comfort, A. (1990) *A Good Age*, Pan Books, London.

Cooper, G.F. (1988) The psychological methods of sex therapy, in Cole, M. and Dryden, W. (eds) *Sex Therapy in Britain*, pp. 127–164, Open University Press, Milton Keynes.

Denny, M.W., Field, J.K. and Quadango, D. (1984) Sex differences in sexual needs and desires, *Archiv. Sex. Behav.*, 13, 233–245.

Engelhardt, H.T. (1974) The disease of masturbation: values and concept of disease, *Bull. Hist. Med.*, 48, 234–248.

Felstein, I. (1986) *Understanding Sexual Medicine*, M.T.P. Press, Lancaster.

Friedman, G.S. (1979) Development of a sexual knowledge questionnaire inventory for elderly persons, *Nurs. Res.*, 28, 372–374.

Gochros, H.L. and Fisher, J. (1980) *Treat Yourself to a Better Sex Life*, Prentice Hall, New York.

Greengross, W. (1982) Sex and physical disability, in Lock, S. (ed.) *Problems in Practice*, pp. 75–78. British Medical Journal, London.

Greengross, W. and Greengross, S. (1989) *Living, Loving and Ageing*, Age Concern, London.

Hawton, K. (1985) *Sex Therapy: A Practical Guide*, Oxford University Press, Oxford.

Hite, S. (1976), *The Hite Report*, Dell, New York.

Hollender, M. (1970) The medical profession and sex in 1900, *Am. J. Obstet. Gynecol.*, 108, 139.

Kaplan, H.S. (1979) *Disorders of Sexual Desire*, Baillière Tindall, London.

Kass, D.J. and Strauss, F.F. (1975) *Sex Therapy at Home*, Simon & Schuster, New York.

Kellett, J. (1989) Sex and the elderly, *British Medical Journal*, 299, 14th October, 934.

London, P. (1978) Sexual behavior, in Reich, W.T. (ed.) *Encyclopedia of Bioethics*, The Free Press, New York.

LoPiccolo, J. (1978) Direct treatment of sexual dysfunction, in LoPiccolo, J. and LoPiccolo, L. (eds) *Handbook of Sex Therapy*, Plenum Press, New York.

181

McCarthy, B.W. (1977) *What You Don't Know About Male Sexuality*, T.W. Crowell, New York.

Masters, W.H. and Johnson, V.E. (1966) *Human Sexual Response*, Little, Brown & Co, Boston.

Palmore, E.B. (1969) Predicting longevity: a follow-up controlling for age, *The Gerontologist*, 9, 247–250.

Pfeiffer, E., Verwoerdt, A. and Wang, H.S. (1968) Sexual behavior in aged men and women, *Archiv. Gen. Psychiat.*, 19, 753–758.

Starr, B.D. (1985) Sexuality and aging, *Ann. Rev. Gerontol.*, 5, 97–126.

Starr, B.D. and Weiner, M.B. (1981) *The Starr-Weiner Report on Sex and Sexuality in the Mature Years*, McGrath, New York.

Stayton, W.R. (1978) The core curriculum: what can be taught and what must be taught, in Rosenzweig, N. and Pearsall, F.P. (eds) *Sex Education for the Health Professional: A Curriculum Guide*, Grune & Stratton, New York.

Sviland, M.A.P. (1978) Helping elderly couples become sexually liberated, in LoPiccolo, J. and LoPiccolo, L. (eds) *Handbook of Sex Therapy*, Plenum Press, New York.

Williams, W. (1986), *Man. Woman, and Sexual Desire*; Williams and Wilkins, Sydney.

World Health Organization (1975), *Education and Treatment in Human Sexuality*, Technical Report No. 572. WHO, Geneva.

# 8

# Health and the quality of life in the later years

This chapter examines the relationship between health in the later decades of life, and the quality of life enjoyed by older people. It is difficult to assess the extent of positive health, both emotional and physical; all we can do is to look at the statistics of disease and disability in relation to age, and the ages at which people die, with the probable causes for their death. Some surveys have asked older people for their subjective assessment of their quality of life, and about their health, and these will be referred to later.

Studies in the Scottish borders by Gruer (1976) and by Isaacs and Neville (1975) revealed that only 7% of people aged over 65 were free from the medical conditions the researchers were concerned with. The most common disabilities were joint disorders (43%) and mental disorders (42%). If these percentages seem very high, it must be pointed out that there was no control group of younger people with whom a comparison might be made as to the stringency of the criteria used. Three or more disorders were found in 60% of the population studied, and 70% had at least one condition that was judged to have a significant effect on their lives, but was unknown to their G.P. This may be compared with a study in Finland (WHO, 1982) in which 33% of people over the age of 65 who were interviewed had some chronic disease, and it was alleged that the prevalence of unmet need was high. The Council of Europe has published a report embracing various European countries concerning the health of elderly people (Council of Europe, 1988), and these statistics from Scotland and Finland are by no means atypical.

According to the General Household Survey of the Office of Population Censuses and Surveys (OPCS, 1989), in 1986 some 'long-standing illness' was reported for 61% of men, and 65% of women over the age of 65. Regarding acute illnesses, in the oldest age group (over 75), 47 days in the year for men, and 61 days for women, were periods during which their activities were restricted. This may be compared with the periods of restriction per annum suffered by all age groups of adults – 23 days for men and 29 days for women. This comparison is less striking than may at first appear, for younger people will have to go to work despite suffering from periodic colds, stomach complaints, and rheumatic attacks, etc., whereas older people, being retired, can afford to rest up at home during such attacks. The above findings may seem rather depressing, but they highlight the fact that the concepts of 'disease' and 'disability' are highly flexible. Writing of the Gothenburg Longitudinal Study of 70-year-olds, Svanborg states the following:

> As far as we can judge, at least 30% and probably 40–50% of the 70-year-olds were at the time of investigation without any symptoms of definable disease. We are still at the present time of our longitudinal study aware of the fact that these figures are minimal and that extended longitudinal experiences might further increase that percentage. As far as we now can judge, there are, at the age of 79, still at least 20% that are obviously healthy. It should be emphasised that among those with definable disease many of the occurring diseases were mild and of such nature that they should not have influenced e.g. the referenced values mentioned in this lecture. Only 5% were suffering from advanced handicap at age 70, 10% at age 75 and 20% at age 79 (Svanborg, 1985, pp. 232–233.).

## THE IMPORTANCE OF SUBJECTIVE WELL-BEING

It is evident that the ideal of perfect health is largely illusory, and that with ageing various systems of the body suffer from the effects of senescence that are either noticed by the people themselves, or are discernable on medical examination. But this does not mean that all the pathological changes and diseases that develop in later life necessarily cause older people to lead miserable lives. It is quite clear that the great majority of people adapt to the changes that take place with ageing right from early adulthood, and may be leading as happy, or happier, lives with their comparatively inefficient bodies, as they did when they were young and fully robust. According to Henwood (1990), 'Despite the objective evidence concerning levels of ill-health and disability in old age, more than 60 per cent of people aged over 65 describe their health as 'good' or 'very good' (p. 45).

What is important for enjoying life is the *subjective* experience of well-being. It is difficult to define just what we mean by 'well-being'; it is an emotional condition and is not dependent on the robustness of the body. Young adults may look at pensioners whose gait has lost its spring, and whose heads are bald or grey, and think, 'Poor old things! I hate to think what is in store for me.' Yet they do not know that many of these older people may be getting more out of life than their young contemporaries, and their sympathy is inappropriate. This curious phenomenon of subjective 'well-being' is quite an important factor. It was discussed in Chapter 3 how studies by Mossey and Shapiro (1982), and others, showed that it was subjectively perceived well-being, more than objectively determined health, that predicted longevity. If people are enjoying life, they will ignore their various age-related disabilities and continue to function as total people pretty well. The other side of the coin is demonstrated by the mortality figures of those recently widowed. Young *et al.* (1963), in a large study involving 4,486 widowers, found that there was a peak of mortality in the first year of bereavement. They found an increase in the death rate of those over 54 of almost 40% during the first six months of bereavement, but after the widowers had apparently got over the acute misery of losing their wives, the death rate dropped off rapidly to that normal for men of their age. Parkes (1986) cites similar data from other studies, and Helsing *et al.* (1981) found that widowers who remarried not only had a mortality rate lower than those who did not, but lower than that of married men who had not been bereaved. The latter finding implies that renewal of a sexual and affectionate relationship has a rejuvenating effect.

## THE CAUSES OF DEATH IN LATER LIFE

All of us must die sometime, but it is encouraging to know that the popular idea of older people deteriorating year after year, until they finally die, is incorrect. Whatever age-related changes

**Table 8.1** Main causes of death in the older age cohorts in 1988. Figures percentaged by column

|  | Age cohorts | | | | | | |
| --- | --- | --- | --- | --- | --- | --- | --- |
| Disease | 55–64 | | 65–74 | | 75–84 | | 85+ | |
| Heart disease | 22,004 | 34.4% | 48,060 | 35.0% | 65,637 | 32.9% | 35,826 | 29.7% |
| Cancer | 25,020 | 39.1 | 44,477 | 32.4 | 43,874 | 22.0 | 14,818 | 12.3 |
| Respiratory | 4,162 | 6.5 | 11,967 | 8.7 | 22,285 | 11.3 | 20,030 | 16.5 |
| Cerebrovascular | 3,816 | 6.0 | 13,017 | 9.4 | 29,217 | 14.7 | 20,263 | 16.8 |
| Other | 8,893 | 14.0 | 19,916 | 14.5 | 37,959 | 19.1 | 29,887 | 24.7 |

Source: Office of Population Censuses and Surveys. (1988) *Mortality Statistics* Series DH2. No. 15, HMSO, London.

in organs and bodily functions are taking place, most individuals continue to function at a fairly even level for many years, until there is a relatively sudden decline in their health and they die. This matter was discussed in Chapter 3 where several references that give relevant findings are cited. If we are to consider when and why people die, the statistics for mortality in England and Wales, as given by the Office of Population Censuses and Surveys (OPCS, 1988), provide some useful information, as set out in Table 8.1.

It will be seen in Table 8.1 that while heart disease accounts for a fairly steady percentage of deaths across all age cohorts, the incidence of death from cancer (expressed as a percentage of the total deaths) steadily diminishes with age. Death from respiratory diseases and from cerebrovascular accidents increases steadily with age, as does the great variety of causes classed as 'other'. This table can be further broken down by sex, and the actual figures reveal that in each age cohort the death rate of men is far higher in relation to the population, than that of women. Such a table may be regarded as an amalgamation of two different tables showing the figures for the two sexes separately. As well as women being more robust in the later years of life, and longer-lived, the pattern of disease in relation to death is rather different, but this matter need not concern us further here.

One of the chief implications of this table is that when considering the population over the age of 54 we are not concerned with just one homogeneous group, but a number of groups whose characteristics are, so far, ill-defined. While some are so vulnerable that they die in their 50s, others are so tenacious of life, whatever their physical disabilities objectively diagnosed, that they live on into their 90s and beyond. We do not know what are the main factors during this span of 40 years that determine long-continued vigour and late death, or to what extent the eventual fate of an individual is largely controlled by the programming in the genetic material.

## LONGEVITY

The search for the secret of longevity, the 'elixir of youth', is a very old one, and we have not space properly to consider its history here. There has always been a belief that longevity was in some way connected with sexuality, and many of the ancient nostrums that were supposed to promote longevity contained material from the sexual organs of animals, as described by Cordellas (1934). One of the first attempts to rejuvenate men in terms of modern medicine was that of Charles Brown-Sequard who injected himself with testicular material from various animals and claimed that it had produced in him renewed vigour and enjoyment of life. This was in 1889 when he was 72 years of age; he died five years later. Experiments with various species with the transplantation of the testes of young animals into the bodies of senile animals convinced some scientists that this would eventually lead to a practical means by which human life could be prolonged. Such work is principally associated with the names of Steinach and Voronoff. Voronoff implanted the testes of monkeys in elderly men and claimed that this did indeed rejuvenate them, but as the experiments were not properly controlled, there was no evidence that it had any effect on their life-span. From what we now know about organ implantation, and the actual effects of the injection of testosterone, it is plain that Voronoff's experiments could have had no relevant physiological effect on his patients, but their status was probably improved by the placebo effect. A review of the work of these two doctors is given by Walton (1929).

Later research into longevity has turned away from such crude physiological experimentation to anthropological and sociological inquiries. This does not mean that physiological research is not relevant and important in the study of geriatrics and gerontology; unquestionably it is, and the steady accumulation of physiological knowledge about ageing processes will certainly pay off in the future, but no quick solutions are to be expected, and we may learn a great deal about ageing and the prospects for the future by studying the life-style and health of human populations in natural settings.

Reports began to accumulate about populations in different parts of the world where many people lived to a very great age and retained their vigour to a far greater extent than is normal in the advanced Western nations. Leaf (1973) studied various communities, including the villagers of Vilcamamba in Ecuador, Hunza in Kashmir, and Abkhazia in the USSR, where it was reputed that many people lived to a great age. He claimed that he had discovered some common denominators of longevity, including no retirement from work, a moderate indulgence in 'vices', a strong sex-drive, fertility in women, and limited calorific intake. Later inquiries have thrown doubt on the information that the people themselves gave to those questioning them, and Leaf himself realized that he had been misled in Ecuador (Leaf, 1978). It is difficult to conduct such inquiries in places where the registration of births a long time ago was not very accurate, and where the people themselves, proud of their reputation, have a motive for exaggerating their age. Various researchers have thrown doubt on the validity of the supposed findings (Rosenwaite and Preston, 1984), and Mazzess and Matheson (1982) have produced evidence that the supposedly long-lived Ecuadorians actually have a life expectancy less than that of the population of the USA.

There is no evidence that any special diet or way of life is particularly productive of a long life; what is more important is a study of the factors that are responsible for early death, factors that we can do something about. The expectation of life for older people, which is a matter different from the general expectation of life for the population, has increased greatly during the present century both due to improvements in public health, and improvement in the medical treatment of conditions such as pneumonia that used to be almost certain killers in the later years of life. Looking at the four major classes of disease that are the main cause of death in the years after the age of 54, as shown in Table

8.1, it is evident that every individual may prolong his or her life by considering the known risks that are associated with these conditions. It has been suggested earlier that genetic programming may predispose us to early or late death, and this idea has considerable scientific support (see Burnet, 1978): thus a man whose genetic predisposition strongly predisposes him to die in the late 60s will be most unlikely to survive into the 90s however careful he is. Nevertheless, by taking sensible measures he may prolong his life quite a few years.

It has been shown that there is some evidence that widowers who re-marry will have longer lives than those who do not, but this does not imply that there is any magic virtue in the sexual relationship. We may go no further than considering a common-sense explanation for this fact. Loneliness, depression and idleness are potential killers because they predispose people to neglect themselves. In an emotional state of misery people tend to indulge too heavily in drinking, eating an inadequate or badly balanced diet, smoking excessively, and taking all sorts of dangerous risks with their health. If they suspect that they have a cancerous growth, they may neglect to have it investigated at an early stage and so die from it. If they are badly housed without adequate warmth in winter, they are less likely to bother to do anything effective about it. They are specially vulnerable. In Table 8.1 the category 'other' covers the deaths by suicide, and they form a percentage that steadily mounts with age, reaching 27 per 100,000 for males of 85 years and over in England and Wales in 1988 (OPCS, 1988). This is almost certainly an under-estimate, as doctors are reluctant to attribute a death to suicide if another cause is plausible. However, this is only the visible tip of the iceberg of men who are despairing of life and longing for death. Men in this unhappy position are hardly likely to take any care of their health, and so will succumb to one of the diseases and hazards to which older people are specially liable, and will die at an earlier age than those who look after themselves properly.

It may be asked why men who have remarried are slightly longer-lived than those who have simply stayed married, and pre-deceased their wives. Although the married state is certainly a protective condition for most men, and enables them to live longer, it is no guarantee of continued appetite for life. The widowed men who re-marry later are likely to be people who show some determination to make the best of the remainder of their lives. All that has been said earlier applies also to women, but to a lesser degree. Women in general are not so badly affected by bereavement as men, at least in terms of their raised mortality; married women live only slightly longer than those who are single, widowed or divorced, and their suicide rate in later life is about a half to a third of that of men of equivalent age.

One very valuable source of information about longevity comes form the longitudinal studies of normal ageing carried out by Duke Univesity in Northern Carolina. From the great mass of evidence produced by this research project, we may turn to that of Palmore (1982) based on the findings of a 25-year follow up. The median age of the population studied was 70 years: 48% were male and 52% female. For the sake of brevity, the brief summary of Palmore's findings related to the indices of longevity that has been prepared by Busse will be quoted:

1. Parents' longevity: The father's age at death was a significant predictor only for men; the mother's age was not.
2. Intelligence: The two components of intelligence, performance and verbal skills, indicated that the verbal performance was a stronger predictor than the preformance. He attributes the strength of intelligence (as a predictor) to 'greater problem-solving ability and better coping mechanisms'.
3. Socioeconomic status: This was a moderate-to-strong predictor for men. This is a not unusual finding as it has been repeatedly demonstrated that high socioeconomic groups enjoy better health and live longer. Although he does not mention it, it also may be related to the intelligence factor.
4. Activity: Locomotor activity was a fairly strong predictor of longevity among the women. This predictor was less so for the more active men. Other types of activity were also looked at, including social club memberships. It is suggested that these activities contribute to one's psychological gratifications. Palmore concludes that, 'All these activity predictors probably relate to the importance of staying active.'
5. Sexual relations: Frequency of intercourse was a significant predictor of longevity for men. For women, this was not necessarily as important, but past enjoyment of intercourse was a significant, moderately strong predictor of longevity.
6. Tobacco and alcohol: Tobacco had a significant negative

relationship. Alcohol was not a significant predictor, but heavy use of alcohol was not frequent in this sample.
7. Satisfactions: Sources of satisfactions were considered. Involvement with religion is not a significant predictor. Men in poorer health and lower economic status have more religious activities than the other males of the group. Work satisfaction and happiness were the strongest predictors.
8. Health: Health is the strongest of the predictor variables (Busse, 1985, pp. 227–228).

It may be noted that the health-measure was *self-rated* health, which may be a better predictor of longevity than objectively rated health, as was noted in Chapter 3, although objective examination by a doctor may discover conditions unknown to the patient.

Most of the more important predictor variables in the Duke University study were concerned with keeping men, the weaker vessels, in reasonable health. Although all the above factors are expressed in positive terms, they might just as well be expressed in negative terms; the predictors of *early death* are early death of the father, lower intelligence and consequent poorer work experience and low pay, loneliness, sexual frustration, excessive smoking, unhappiness and lack of work satisfaction, and finally *self-rated* ill-health. It is perhaps more important for health-care workers to view the problem in these negative terms, for they are primarily concerned with helping the casualties of society. However, it appears that the best means of maximizing the potential for health and longevity in the later years of life does not lie with any one factor, but with the general promotion of the quality of life. If older people are happy, occupied and possessed of a true sense of their own value and dignity, they will look after themselves and be less likely to become a burden on the medical and social services.

The strange finding that for men frequency of sexual intercourse was a significant positive predictor of longevity, but for women this was 'not necessarily as important, but past enjoyment of intercourse was a significant, moderately strong predictor of longevity', deserves some comment. This was a 25-year follow-up study, and as it progressed many more of the men died off leaving their wives widowed and unable to enjoy any sex lives, at least, as far as heterosexual intercourse went. But for both sexes, sexuality was a positive predictor. Here we cannot distinguish between cause and effect. Does the expression of sexualty in itself promote health and longevity, as was believed by the ancients who prepared allegedly potent nostrums, or is active sexuality just one of the manifestations of continued physical and emotional health? To date we just do not know, and although some of the work in endocrinology is suggestive, the question remains unanswered.

## SOME COMMON DISABILITIES IN RELATION TO THE QUALITY OF LIFE

### Hypochondriasis

Conditions of hypochondriasis are likely to develop in later life, and although they are not in themselves either life-threatening or productive of serious disability, they do seriously detract from the quality of life experienced by many older people, and cause a good deal of extra work for health-care workers. The term hypochondriasis has a very ancient history, and a somewhat chequered status in modern times in medical diagnosis. As it is currently used, its definition appears in the revised third edition of the *Diagnostic and Statistical Manual of Mental Disorders* (American Psychiatric Association, 1987). It may simply be defined as an anxious preoccupation with one's own body, or a particular part of the body, which is believed to be either diseased or seriously malfunctioning, in the absence of adequate evidence. An otherwise reasonable person may hold quite extraordinary delusions about a supposed pathological condition despite medical assurance that there is nothing wrong. It can, of course, be associated with an actually paranoid psychotic condition, (Munro, 1980) but it is generally a monosymptomatic neurosis indicating a difficulty in adjusting to ageing (Busse and Pfeiffer, 1977). Molière's play, *Le Malade Imaginaire*, depicts such a sufferer, and it is alleged that Molière himself was hypochondriacal (Turner *et al.*, 1984). The condition is not confined to older people, but it is likely to intensify in later life. In Lipsett's (1970) study of hypochondriacal patients it was found that most of them were female and over the age of 58. Bianchi

(1971) reported that the most usual hypochondriacal delusions concerned cancer (47%) and heart failure (30%), and this is very understandable because so many older people have friends and relatives who die of these two diseases.

Although health-care workers should be fully aware of the nature of hypochondriasis in later life, all complaints must be taken seriously for two reasons. There is always the possibility of some physical disease underlying the complaint, although not necessarily that which the patient fears. It is a nuisance constantly to be requesting medical investigations when there are no reasonable grounds for suspecting that there is anything to be discovered, but there is always the chance that something may have been missed. In one sense, it is better for patients to be over-concerned about their health in later life and demand investigation, than to neglect themselves until a serious condition has developed. The other reason why hypochondriacal complaints must receive careful and sympathetic consideration is that although the manifest complaints may be delusory and even absurd, the patients are trying to tell the doctor or other health-care professional something about themselves which is important and which needs treatment. When the patient has been reassured again and again that there is absolutely no sign of cancer of the bowel, the doctor must consider what is really wrong with the patient in a psycho-social sense, and to what kind of health-care professional he or she should be referred. This may seem the most elementary common sense, but in view of the huge amounts of placative drugs that continue to be prescribed and consumed by older people, it does not seem to be universally followed.

It is tempting to take the view that some people are just inveterate complainers, and that their hypochondriasis is a manifestation of a fundamental personality trait. This does not appear to be the case, however, and hypochondriasis may be relatively temporary and resulting from a transient situation. In the Duke University study that has already been referred to, as there were repeated investigations of the same people over quite a long span of years, it was discovered that hypochondriacal reactions came and went according to the life circumstances of people studied. When the quality of their life was good, quite irrespective of their general health, they were free from such reactions, but when adverse psycho-social circumstances developed, they would begin to notice minor aches and pains and project their worries and fears on some physical system. With a fortuitous alleviation of stress, the hypochondriacal preoccupation would disappear. For the first six rounds of observations a rating of hypochondriasis was made, and continued observation showed that there was no constant tendency in the same people. There was no consistent pattern of association of this tendency with sex, race, physical health, nearness to death, or financial condition. The only variable with which it was consistently associated was depression. At the final analysis of the data it was found that over half the 'survivors', (those alive and still available for study after 25 years), had received a diagnosis of hypochondriasis at some time or other, which tells us something about the prevalence of this condition in later life.

## Depression

The traditional picture of depression in older people is rather a grim one, and when an elderly member of a family succumbs to a depressive illness, the relatives sometimes tend to wonder if he or she had 'gone mad' or 'gone senile', both labels implying that a permanent pathological change has taken place in their relative. The view of clinical depression in later life that is traditionally held by professional people is not much better. The clinical picture is supposed to display features which include agitation, behaviour that is paranoid, or extremely withdrawn and obsessive-compulsive. It is held that the prognosis for recovery is rather poor, and this gloomy forecast may be unintentionally conveyed to the relatives.

A number of studies have contributed to this picture (e.g. Goldstein, 1979; Post, 1972; Roth, 1976; Saltzman and Shader; Steur et al., 1980), and the implication is that degenerative processes in the brain and the whole physiological system are responsible for intractable depression in later life. According to Millard (1983) 'no matter what is done, a third get better, a third stay the same, and a third get worse.' Thus there seems to be no real hope for two thirds of the older depressive sufferers.

Some more recent studies have called into question the classic picture of depression in elderly people. Studies such as those of Baldwin (1988), Baldwin and Jolley (1986), Benbow (1989), Musetti et al. (1990), have indicated that depression in later life is neither so serious nor so chronic as has generally been assumed, and that it is sometimes more easily treated than the depressions that affect the population under the age of 60.

There are wide variations in the estimates of the incidence of depressive illnesses among people over 60 living in the community. Baldwin and Jolley (1986) suggest 11–12%, Coni et al. suggest 10–15%, Gianturco and Busse (1978) give 21.5% for the elderly population they studied, Heckenheimer (1989) indicates that 10–65% of older people experience depression, and Haggerty et al. (1988) gives an incidence of 10–20%. It seems that all assessors have not been using the same criteria when they use the term.

Gurland (1976) makes a distinction between 'Depression *as diagnosed by psychiatrists*', and as established by '*symptoms* not necessarily assessed by psychiatrists' – the prevalence of which have been assessed in large-scale population studies. The incidence of the former appears to be greatest in the middle years of life, but the latter appears to be more prevalent in the later years. He concludes that:

> on the whole, the majority of definite depressive disorders appear to occur before the age of 65. Nevertheless, this should not distract from the high prevalence of depression after the age of 65 years with short-term rates of about 2% to 3% for severe depressions and up to 3% to 4% for definite but mild depressions (Gurland, 1976, p. 290).

The diagnositic criteria given in the four successive editions of the *Diagnostic and Statistical Manual of Mental Disorders* have gradually clarified the concept. The most recent revised edition (DSM III-R, American Psychiatric Association, 1987) gives a somewhat complex classification, but broadly, depressive illnesses can be categorized as biploar or unipolar types, the former exhibiting the well-known swing between depressive and manic phases, but the latter returning to normal after the depressive episode is over. The biploar type is sometimes known as 'endogenous (psychotic) depression', and the unipolar type 'reactive (neurotic) depression'. One might expect that the depressions of later life would be predominantly of the biologically determined endogenous type, the result of physiological deterioration, as suggested by Post (1972) and Jacoby (1981), but more recent evidence indicates the contrary. Evidence has been accumulating by studies comparing depressed people, say below the age of 60, with those whose first episodes of depression have occurred after that age, such as those of Benbow (1989), Burvill *et al.* (1989), Musetti *et al.* (1989). In the study of Musetti and her colleagues, 400 patients with major depression were divided into two groups, those above and below the age of 65, and compared over a wide range of characteristics. They report that:

> In the present study which focused on a consecutive and very large sample of patients with rigorously defined primary major depression, neither chronicity nor inter-episodic residuals, were related to old age. It is possible that the clinical picture of greater chronicity of depression in old age is derived from in-patient or clinical samples in which depressions have been mixed with other psychiatric and physical disorders. . . . bipolar I and bipolar II disorders and recurrent (unipolar) depression typically arise before age 65 and show high familial prevalence of mood disorders; this is particularly true for the bipolar I type characterized by mania. Single-episode depression, by contrast, was significantly more common after age 65; environmental factors, such as stressors identified within six months of the onset of depression, were more common in this sub-type (Musetti *et al.*, 1989, pp. 334–335).

These findings imply that while elderly people are less likely to be subject to endogenous psychotic depression, their depressive episodes are more frequently the direct result of environmental stressors. When the impact of such stressors has been overcome, the patient recovers from the depression. The major stressors of later life include retirement, alteration in health status, bereavement, adjustment to a new role in society, and in some cases, real poverty.

This summary may tend to over-simplify what is really a very complex matter, and diagnosis of the type of depression from which anyone is suffering must be left to specialists. However, such an interpretation of the broad facts about depression in later life serves to caution health-care workers against accepting the traditional and highly pessimistic attitude towards depression in older people that was common a little while ago.

The findings of the study by Musetti *et al.* are largely confirmed by those of Emerson *et al.* (1989), although the latter authors found that it was men, rather than women, whose depressive episodes appeared to be more directly due to stressful life events. Not only do these and other recent research studies present a more hopeful picture of the nature of depression in later life, but they give us reason to be energetic in seeing that people get prompt treatment. Baldwin and Jolley (1986) studied 100 people aged 65–88 who were so seriously depressed that they had to be admitted to hospital. In the year before admission, 79% of them had suffered a major stressful situation, and 18 of them had actually attempted suicide. Antidepressant medication had previously been given to 47% of them, but without improvement. With regard to treatment in hospital, 45% were given antidepressant drugs, and 48% had electroconvulsive therapy (ECT), sometimes in conjunction with drugs. After treatment in hospital, 20 were able to return home in less than a month, and 56 before 3 months. Only 3 remained for more than a year. In view of modern criticisms of ECT, this may seem a high proportion of elderly patients to receive such treatment, but there is now evidence that older people respond better to ECT than do younger (Benbow, 1989), and according to Baldwin (1988), 'The advent of ECT dramatically improved the outcome for old people with severe depression. Where depression does persist, it becomes associated with somatic problems.'

When older people have broken down into a depressive illness, health-care workers should not only provide a rescue service by referring them for proper treatment, and reassuring them and their families about the likelihood of complete recovery, but also they should serve a preventive function. For if they succeed in helping to maintain the quality of older people's lives in various ways, they will be less vulnerable to the stressors of later life that cause such breakdowns.

### Dementia, pseudodementia, and confusion

Bernard Ineichen (1989) illustrates the first page of his book on dementia with a cartoon showing two figures who are presumably social workers. One of them is saying to the other, 'Senile dementia? Isn't that when elderly clients disagree with you about what's best for them?' This pretty well illustrates the common over-use of the term dementia.

Bennet (1989) suggests that about one in ten of the population over the age of 65, and one in five of those over 85, have some form of dementia, but he admits that, 'The most recent work done in this field suggests that may be an over-estimate.' It is very difficult to obtain reliable information retrospectively about the incidence of dementia in relation to age, since the onset of the condition is usually insidious. This indicates that among the 'young old' there may be many in whom a dementing illness has begun to develop, but they may die from other causes before the condition is detected. Roth (1978) conducted a five-year follow-up survey of a random sample of people living in Newcastle on Tyne, and estimated that there was an annual incidence of senile or arteriosclerotic dementia of 1.4% among people over the age of 65. This is not significantly different from the annual incidence of 2.3% among those over 60 reported by Hagnell (1966) in Sweden, because the latter figure was somewhat swollen by the inclusion of other psychiatric cases.

Dementia is caused by neural degeneration or injury. As defined in the DSMIII-R, it involves global loss of cognitive function, and shows in loss of memory, defective judgement, impaired comprehension, and loss of the ability to think in abstract terms. There are two main types of dementia in elderly people: (i) primary degenerative dementia, the most common type being Alzheimer's disease, which results from neural degeneration (SDAT – senile dementia of the Alzheimer type); (ii) multi-infarct dementia (MID) caused by many small infarcts in cortical and sub-cortical areas, and it is sometimes accompanied by motor and sensory changes.

In SDAT the deterioration is slow and gradual, but MID is characterized by quite sudden changes interspersed with periods of stability, as the degeneration proceeds in a step-wise fashion. The two types occur with about equal frequency up to the mid 80s, after which the SDAT becomes about six times as common, because so many MID cases have died. Wattis (1984) gives the 13 points of the weighted Hachinski scoring system on which a classic case of MID can score the maximum of 18 points. A score of over 7 indicates that the patient is probably a MID case, and below 4 indicates SDAT.

In an elderly person who is dementing, there may be various processes contributing to the condition, such as myxoedema, vitamin B12 deficiency, alcoholism, chronic sub-dural haematoma, normal-pressure hydrocephalus, instead of, or in addition to, the two main conditions described above. It is therefore necessary to attempt as precise a diagnosis as possible, because some of the factors may be reversible and call for appropriate action by health-care workers. It is unwise to assume that this is just another Alzheimer case, despite the appearance of all the classic features.

One of the reasons why dementia in later life may be over-diagnosed is the possibility that it is really pseudodementia. Haggerty *et al.* (1989) estimate that in 10–15% of cases diagnosed as demented, there is no organic disorder but the symptoms mimic a true dementia. Such cases are generally remediable and the patients can be returned to full cognitive functioning if the condition is detected and treated appropriately. This is, of course, of great importance for the individual, the family, and for social policy, for if the true condition remains undetected, an elderly person may be left to vegetate in a residential institution, or in a back room of a family home, when he or she could be restored to living a full and independent life.

The question arises, why should some people appear to lose their memories, the power to think clearly, and the ability to look after themselves, when there is really nothing at all wrong with their brains? Haggerty *et al.* note that:

> Patients with pseudodementia often demonstrate impaired motivation and energy when responding to questions – questions are answered with 'I don't know' or 'I don't remember' – and there is little effort to conceal intellectual deficits through confabulation or avoidance. In fact, at times it will appear that these patients highlight and exaggerate the degree and importance of their deficits. By contrast, demented patients frequently deny their cognitive deficits (Haggerty *et al.*, 1989, p. 65).

That people should act as though they were hopelessly demented when they are not, and when such a presentation of themselves generally results in their being housed and cared for in the most dreary settings, may seem very strange. Their condition is generally the result of a major depression, and in the view of Wells (1979) one of the most striking features of such patients is a long-standing tendency to depend upon others for physical care and emotional support even before their breakdown. They wish to become helpless, and to accentuate their helplessness, at whatever cost to themselves.

Although we can explain pseudodementia in terms of a deep depression bringing on a sense of worthlessness and a desire to be utterly taken care of, such an explanation does not rule out the possibility of pseudodementia co-existing with some degree of true dementia. True dementia may also co-exist with major depression. According to Cummings (1987), from 5–20% of Alzheimer cases, and 25–30% of multi-infarct cases have concurrent depression. It is of interest that in a study by Reiffler *et al.* (1987), while depression was found in 20–30% of patients with mild or moderate degrees of dementia, among the patients with really severe degrees of dementia the incidence of depression was only 12%. This suggests that in the early stages of dementia patients tend to know what is happening to them, and this experience may be profoundly depressing for then, but later on they lose touch with reality to the extent that they are not specially concerned.

Because depression, dementia, and pseudodementia may all occur together in different combinations, the task of accurate diagnosis is one for specialists. However, all health-care workers should be fully aware of the possible complications and, according to their different disciplines, be prepared to co-operate in the task of gathering relevant information from different sources – from the patients themselves, the family, all the professional care agencies – that will contribute to an accurate diagnosis. It may be that some people with an apparently hopeless degree of depressive withdrawal or advanced dementia, can be restored to full or partial independence.

'Is the patient confused or demented?' This is the title of an excellent article by Wattis (1984). He points out that the confused patient rarely makes contact with professional sources of care, and it is left to the worried families or the neighbours to report that something may be wrong. Obviously, home visiting is the most important way of detecting a confused state. Elderly people may become confused, but appear to be demented, as the result of a temporary illness. Infections of the chest or urinary system, heart trouble, alcoholic withdrawal, dietary deficiency, and other physiological disturbances may all cause an acute confusional state in otherwise normal elderly people. If there is already some degree of dementia, very minor upsets of a transient nature such as a change of home or constipation may bring on acute confusion. It is unfortunate that confused elderly patients cannot be relied on to take the steps necessary for their rehabilitation, such as taking medication or reforming their diet, so if they normally live alone they will need to be admitted to hospital or go to stay with a relative until they are better. The confused person will often feel bewildered and frightened and unable to remember who a health-care worker is, so repeated re-orientation may be necessary, such as saying, 'I am your social worker and I have come again to . . .'

It is heartening to bear in mind that many confused elderly people can be restored to normality and independence given the right treatment, and that even when there is a mild degree of dementia present, when the confused state has cleared up, most elderly demented people can live at home, and only about one in eight needs to be in institutional care.

## Insomnia

Many older people complain of insomnia and believe that their health is being adversely affected by lack of sleep. Fortunately, it is a condition which health-care professionals can often alleviate or abolish simply by giving sound advice. First, we must consider precisely what is meant by insomnia. Some writers make statements such as, 'in old age it has been estimated that at least 50 per cent of people suffer from insomnia' (Zarit, 1980, p. 233), and such statements are pretty meaningless unless the term 'insomnia' is precisely defined. Insomnia may be usefully defined as *a condition in which sufferers feel that they do not get enough sleep, and are distressed by the subjectively experienced lack of it.*

The main difference that normal ageing makes to sleep is that stage 4 sleep, the deepest level, becomes less and less, so that by about the age of 60 it may become totally eliminated, and EEG studies of the sleeping brain show that the deepest level reached is stage 3 (Hayashi and Endo, 1982). Older people tend to awaken more during the night; the number of their awakenings at age 60 is nearly three times that at age 20 (Kales and Kales, 1984). Older people should therefore be told that as there is nothing pathological about their changing patterns of sleep, they have no need to worry.

As, by our definition, insomnia is a condition of *believing* that not enough sleep is being obtained, and there is subjective distress because of such belief and the associated experience, we may refer to some people as 'insomniacs' whether or not they sleep much or little. If we compare younger with older insomniacs, we find a most interesting difference. The younger people tend to recognize that their insomnia is mainly due to their anxiety, depression, and emotional problems, whereas older people tend to deny this, and to insist that their sleeplessness is due to various physical conditions. As found by Kales *et al.* (1976), older people tend to blame what they have had for supper, noises in the street, the temperature of the room, an uncomfortable bed, etc., in order to avoid facing the fact that their inability to get to sleep, or to stay asleep, is due to emotional problems. Why this age-related difference exists is something of a mystery; conditions of pain and sickness that are more common in later life do, of course, disrupt sleep, but in the absence of such definite disorders, the stressors are likely to be psychological whatever the age of the person.

What is happening with ageing is that the 24-hour sleep-wakefulness cycle that is established in early childhood is becoming disrupted, with an increasing tendency to revert to the multi-phase pattern of sleep that characterizes infancy. Many older people show a tendency to take day-time naps, partly as a result of this disruption of the 24-hour cycle, and because of such napping their sleep at night becomes more fitful. Those complaining of insomnia should therefore be advised to try to resist the day-time naps in order to maintain the 24-hour cycle as far as is possible. Taking day-time naps is sometimes due to boredom, and they will be less desired if people live busier and more stimulating lives. It may be said that while it is easy to advise a 'busier and more stimulating life', it is less easy to achieve such a goal. However, it is essential that people complaining of insomnia should be instructed in the realities of the situation, and not be left to wonder if there is something organically wrong with them. While a satisfactory sex-life does not guarantee an acceptable pattern of sleep, a frustrated sex-life may well be at the root of insomnia, and Butler and Lewis (1988) advise that, 'Active, pleasurable sexual activity, including sexual self-stimulation, can be an excellent sleep inducer. This effect is strongest when there is orgasm, but even without it such activity is usually relaxing.'

Although idiopathic insomnia is not a serious health problem, the complaint must be treated seriously, and a proper investigation made as it may be a symptom of some pathological condition such as clinical depression, neurological dysfunctions (sleep apnoea or nocturnal myoclonus), or drug abuse. Assuming that there is no underlying pathology, then some insomnia will clear up completely when the patient is brought to an understanding of sleep, and a re-assessment of the whole problem. Patients should be confronted with the fact that they may not *need* any more sleep than they are getting. Due sympathy should be shown for their understandable distress, but the distress may be caused not by insufficient sleep, but by the hours spent in struggling to get to sleep, with all the associated anxiety and the black, depressive thoughts that come in the wakeful small hours. Individual differences in the need for sleep are enormous, and a difference of five to nine hours sleep a night is quite within the normal range. If a person whose natural need for sleep is about five hours a night believes that eight hours is necessary, then that person is suffering from insomnia. Such researchers as Horne (1988), Meddis (1977), and Stuss and Broughton (1978), have investigated just why people vary so much in their need for sleep, but there seem to be no important ways in which short-sleepers differ from long-sleepers.

Unfortunately, there are many cheap books on the market advising people on how to get a better night's sleep without pointing out that some short-sleepers do not require any more sleep and are worrying unnecessarily. Kevin Morgan comments that:

the commonly held belief that eight hours sleep is a universal norm for adult human beings also does little to prepare anyone for the declining total sleep time so characteristic of growing old. This particular item of mis-information can pop up in the most incongruous places. For example, in an otherwise helpful book intended for those 'Caring for an elderly relative', Dr Keith Thompson asserts that 'Most people need about seven or eight hours' sleep a night.' Most young people might, most elderly people certainly *do not* (Morgan, 1987, p. 141).

Morgan goes on to discuss the medical response to complaints of insomnia, and asserts that the prescription of hypnotic drugs is the principal and often the only medical way of dealing with insomnia, whether the patient is young, middle-aged, or elderly. Medical attitudes to the prescription of hypnotic drugs has changed in more recent years. Oswald and Adams (1983) cite a large Scottish survey in which nearly 45% of all the women over 75 took sleeping drugs. What doctors have been prescribing such drugs for is not really to increase sleep because the patients need it, but to combat the dreadful experience of anxiety and depression that accompanies the hours of wakefulness when the insomniac is worrying about being unable to sleep and reviewing the whole of his or her life in the blackest of terms, perhaps wondering if suicide might be a better alternative to this regularly repeated calvary.

Benzodiazepine drugs once seemed to be a solution to this widespread problem, but now the medical profession is well aware of the bitter harvest from this pharmacological approach. Higgit et al. (1985) review the whole question of benzodiazepine dependence, and conclude that, 'Benzodiazepines should not be prescribed for normal people at times of acute stress such as bereavement or divorce, and a recent study found brief counselling by general practitioners to be as effective as benzodiazepines in cases of minor affective disorder.' They do not refer to insomnia specifically, although this is one of the worst results of such stressful events. Their advice would seem to mean that if the G.P., (once having screened the elderly patient for pathological conditions) is not needed in the key role of drug-prescriber, then other specialists in health-care have an equal role to play in providing the broad spectrum of care that comes under the heading of counselling.

Higgitt et al. provide a number of references to non-pharmacological approaches which can take the place of drug prescription, and Morgan (1987) in his *Sleep and Ageing* devotes a chapter to alternatives to hypnotic drugs.


**Deafness**

This is a most important problem of the later years, for it is far more common than is supposed, and has grave social consequences that should be appreciated by all health-care professionals.

About 5% of people over the age of 50, and 29% of those

over 65, suffer from some degree of hearing loss (Comfort, 1989). Unfortunately, older people have been made ashamed to reveal that they suffer from this handicap, and hence may go to considerable lengths to conceal it, pretending to understand questions when they do not. Professional people may therefore get the impression that their elderly clients are a little stupid and perhaps dementing, when all that is wrong is the professionals not speaking loudly and clearly enough to be properly understood. More educated people generally have the social assurance to ask nurses, doctors and other care-givers to speak up when they talk too softly or mumble, but older people of more humble status may feel that this would be rude. Nowadays it is generally held that to laugh at cripples because of their handicap is very distasteful, but the partial deafness of elderly people is still a permissible subject for humour. The following appears on a matchbox sold by Bryant & Mays:

First old lady. 'Isn't it windy?'
Second old lady. 'No, I think it's Thursday.'
Third old lady. 'So am I. Let's have a cup to tea.'

It is little wonder then that many older people do not like to admit that they have some difficulty in hearing, and they dislike wearing hearing aids even when they have no reluctance to wear spectacles.

The wearing of a hearing aid is not, of course, an invariable remedy, for some forms of inability to hear acutely are due to the condition of tinnitus. The latter condition is very complex and has only recently come in for much study (Hallam, 1989; Slater and Terry, 1987; Youngson, 1986). It presents two problems: some people are driven frantic by the constant experience of ringing and other head noises which affect their mental health; others do not seem to mind the head-noises much, but the distracting subjective noise makes it difficult for them to hear very well, particularly under conditions where there is a good deal of ambient sound. Various remedies such as instruments producing a masking sound are of some use where the person is seriously disturbed by the constant noise, but for the second problem of impaired acuity of hearing there is no adequate remedy, as hearing aids simply magnify the volume of sound, which is not the whole problem. About the best measure to be adopted is for sufferers to ask their friends and family to speak clearly, as well as loudly enough, to be understood. It is this factor of clarity of speech that tends to generate ageist prejudice against elderly people, and cause younger persons to mock their impaired hearing, for many people do not like to be reminded of their slovenly manner of speech, and to be asked to speak more intelligibly.

The problem of impaired hearing in later life is so common that older people, particularly those who often foregather with their age peers, unconsciously learn to speak a little louder and to enunciate their words more precisely than younger people. This is very noticeable at conferences where there is a wide range of ages. Patrick Rabbitt, who has done extensive research with older people and paid particular attention to the question of declining acuity of hearing, observes that:

Hearing loss makes prolonged conversations more effortful and less rewarding. To be stuck with a garrulous bore is bad enough if you have perfect hearing, but if you also have to struggle to follow banalities your legitimate self-defence may gain you attributions of undesirable personality characteristics. For people with slight hearing-loss, the effort of following a long, dull lecture may become so unendurable that blatant inattention or even public dozing is unavoidable. Presbyacusis, which becomes increasingly common in old age, may markedly affect social life by constraining the *environments* in which conversations are possible. A person who can be a lively companion in a quiet room may have to fall silent in aeroplanes and noisy restaurants. Most environments designed for human 'fun' impose severe social constraints on the presbyacusic (Rabbitt, 1988, p. 502).

It may be observed, therefore, that much of the traditional mythology about how older people tend to withdraw from life and become solitary, morose and self-centred, has got nothing to do with any real change in their personalities, but is simply an adaptive modification of habit that is forced on them by the deterioration in the acuity of their hearing.

As so many older people do not wish to admit to this particular handicap because society has made them ashamed of it, it is up to professional care-givers to inquire about their hearing, and not wait to be asked, just as doctors should ask about their sexual function along with other bodily functions. So simple a procedure as syringing the accumulated wax from their ears can have a significant effect on many people's hearing, yet so insidious is the gradual loss of acuity of hearing that many people do not realize that they need it. Similarly, many older people who could benefit from hearing aids have not the initiative to arrange to get them, although they are free under the NHS. According to Comfort (1989), only 400,000 out of 1,300,000 deaf people over 65 have them.

## CONCLUSION

The general subject of the health of older people has been discussed in this chapter, and it is apparent that the quality of life they achieve is of immense importance whatever disabilities have accrued during the passing years. Longevity has been shown to be promoted by the enjoyment of life; avoidance of the major age-related disorders that lead to dangerous ill-health and incapacity is directly related to the sort of emotional adjustment that people are able to make during the process of ageing. Health-care professionals should realize that their duty does not simply lie in providing a rescue service when something goes wrong, but in promoting positive vigour and enjoyment, and that energy and resources devoted to this aim will probably prove most cost-effective in the long run.

## REFERENCES

American Psychiatric Association (1987) *Diagnostic and Statistical Manual of Mental Disorders: Revised*, A.P.A., Washingston, D.C.

Baldwin, R.C. and Jolley, D.J. (1986) The prognosis of depression in old age, *Br. J. Psychiat.*, 149, 574–583.

Benbow, S.M. (1989) The role of electroconvulsive therapy in the treatment of depressive illness in old age, *Br. J. Psychiat.*, 155, 147–152.

Baldwin, R. (1988), Depression in late life: a fresh challenge to an old problem, in Murphy, E. and Parker, S.W. (eds) *Affective Disorders in the Elderly*, pp. 18–27, Churchill Livingstone, Edinburgh.

Benet, G. (1989) *Alzheimer's Disease and Other Confusional States*, McDonald Optima, London.

Bianchi, G. (1971), Patterns of hypochondriasis: a principal component analysis, *Br. J. Psychiat.* 122, 541–548.

Burnet, M. (1978), *Endurance of Life: The Implications of Genetics for Human Life*, Cambridge University Press, Cambridge.

Burvill, P.V., Hall, W.D., Stampfer, H.G. and Emerson, J.P. (1989), A comparison of early-onset and late-onset depressive illness in the elderly, *Br. J. Psychiat.* 155, 673–679.

Busse, E.W. (1985) Normal aging: the Duke Longitudinal studies, in Bergener, M., Ermine, M. and Stanalin, H.B. (eds) *Thresholds of Aging*, Academic Press, London.

Busse, E.W. and Pfeiffer, E. (1977) Introduction, in Busse, E.W. and Pfeiffer, E. (eds) *Behavior and Adaptation in Late Life* 2nd edn, pp. 1–9. Little, Brown & Co, Boston.

Butler, R.N. and Lewis, M.I. (1988) *Love and Sex After 60*, Harper & Row, New York.

Codellas, P.S. (1934) Rejuvenations and satyricons of yesterday, *Ann. Med. History*, 6, 510–520.

Comfort, A. (1989), *A Good Age*, Pan Books, London.

Coni, N, Davison, W. and Webster, S. (1988), *Lecture Notes on Geriatrics*, Blackwell Scientific Publications, Oxford.

Council of Europe (1988) *Surveillance and Screening Techniques for the Elderly*, European Health Committee, Strasbourg.

Cummings, J.L. (1987), Multi-infarct dementia: Diagnosis and management, *Psychosomatics*, 28, 117–126.

Emmerson, J.P., Burvill, P.W., Finlay-Jones, R. and Hall, W. (1989) Life events, life difficulties and confiding relationships in the depressed elderly, *Br. J. Psychiat.*, 155, 787–792.

Gianturco, G.T. and Busse, E., W. (1978) Psychiatric problems encountered during a long-term study of normal aging volunteers, in Isaacs, A.D. and Post, F. (eds) *Studies in Geriatric Medicine*, pp. 1–16. J. Wiley, Chichester.

Goldstein, S.E. (1979) Depression in the elderly, *J. Am. Geriat. Soc.* 27, 38–42.

Gruer, R. (1975) *Needs of the Elderly in the Scottish Borders*, Scottish Health Service Studies, No. 33.

Gurland, B. (1976) The comparative frequency of depression in various adult age groups, *J. Gerontol.*, 31, 283–292.

Haggerty, J.J. Jnr., Golden, R.N., Evans, D.L. and Janowsky D.S. (1988) Differential diagnosis of pseudodementia in the elderly, *Geriatrics*, 43, 61–74.

Hagnell, O. (1966) *A Prospective Study of the Incidence of Mental Disorder*, Svenska Bokfordaget, Stockholm.

Hallam, R. (1989) *Living With Tinnitus*, Thorsons, London.

Hayashi, Y. and Endo, S. (1982) All-night sleep polygraphic recordings of healthy aged persons: REM and slow-wave sleep, *Sleep*, 5, 277–283.

Heckenheimer, E.F. (1989) *Health Promotion of the Elderly in the Community*, W.B. Saunders, Philadelphia.

Helsing, K.J., Szklo, M. and Comstock, G.W. (1981) Factors Associated with mortality, *Am. J. Pub. Health*, 71, 802–809.

Henwood, M. (1990) No sense of urgency: age discrimination in health care, in McEwan, E. (ed.) *Age: The Unrecognized Discrimination*, Age Concern, Mitcham.

Higgitt, A.C., Lader, M.H. and Fonagy, P. (1985) Clinical management of benzodiazepine dependence, *British Medical Journal*, 291, 688–690.

Horne, J. (1988) *Why We Sleep*, Oxford University Press, Oxford.

Ineichen, B. (1989) *Senile Dementia: Policy and Services*, Chapman & Hall, London.

Isaacs, B. and Neville, Y. (1975) *The Measurement of Need in Old People*, Scottish Health Service Studies No. 34.

Jacoby, R.J. (1981) Dementia, depression and the CT scan, *Psychol. Med.*, 11, 673–676.

Kales, A., Caldwell, A.B., Preston, T.A., Healey, S. and Kales, J.D. (1976), Personality patterns in insomnia, *Arch. gen. Psychiat.*, 33, 1128–1134.

Kales, A. and Kales, J.D. (1984) *Evaluation and Treatment of Insomnia*, Oxford University Press, Oxford.

Leaf, A. (1973) Unusual longevity: the common denominators. *Hospital Practice*, October. 74–86.

Leaf, A. (1978) High hoax: the not-so-old Ecuadorians, *Time*, March 27, 87–88.

Lipsett, D.R. (1970) Medical and psychological characteristics of 'crocks', *Psychiat. in Med.*, 1, 15–25.

Mazzess, R.B. and Matheson, R.W. (1982) Lack of unusual longevity in Villacamba, Ecuador, *Hum. Biol.*, 54, 517–524.

Meddis, R. (1977) *The Sleep Instinct*, Routledge & Kegan Paul, London.

Millard, P.H. (1983) Depression in old age, *Br. Med. J.*, 287, 375–376.

Morgan, K. (1987) *Sleep and Ageing*, Croom Helm, London.

Mossey, J.M. and Shapiro, E. (1982) Self-rated health: a predictor of mortality among the aged, *Am. J. Pub. Health*, 72, 800–808.

Munro, A. (1980) Monosymptomatic hypochonriacal psychosis (MPH): new aspects of an old syndrome, *J. Psychiat. Treat. Eval.*, 2, 79.

Musetti, L., Perugi, G., Soriani, A., Rossi, V.M., Cassano, G.B. and Akiskal, H.S. (1989) Depression before and after age 65: a re-examination, *Br. J. Psychiat.*, 155, 330–336.

Office of Population Censuses and Surveys (1988) *Mortality Statistics* Series DH2, No. 15, HMSO, London.

Office of Population Censuses and Surveys (1989) *General Household*, HMSO, London.

Oswald, I. and Adams, K. (1983) *Get A Better Night's Sleep*, Martin Dunitz, London.

Palmore, E.B. (1982) Prediction of the longevity differences: a 25-year follow-up, *The Gerontologist*, 22, 513–518.

Parkes, C.M. (1986) *Bereavement: Studies in Grief in Adult Life*, Penguin Books, Harmondsworth.

Post, F. (1972) The management and nature of depressive illnesses in late life: a follow-through study, *Br. J. Psychiat.*, 1321, 393–404.

Rabbitt, P. (1988) Social psychology, neurosciences and cognitive psychology need each other, (and gerontology needs all three of them). *The Psychologist*, 12,500–506.

Reiffler, B.V., Larson, E. and Hanley, R. (1982) Co-existence of cognitive impairment and depression in geriatric outpatients, *Am. J. Psychiat.*, 139, 623–626.

Rosenwaite, I, and Preston, S.H. (1984) Age-overstatement and Puerto-Rican longevity, *Hum. Biol.*, 53, 503–505.

Roth, M. (1976) The psychiatric disorders of late life, *Psychiat. Annals* 6, 57–101.

Roth, M. (1978) Epidemiological studies, in Katzman, R., Terry, R.D. and Bick, K.L. (eds) *Alzheimer's Disease: Senile Dementia and Related Disorders.* pp. 337–339, Raven Press, New York.

Saltzman, C. and Shader, R.I. (1978) Depression in the elderly, I. Relationship between depression, psychologic defense mechanism and physical illness, *J. Am. Geriat. Soc.*, 26, 253–260.

Slater, R. and Terry, M. (1987) *Tinnitus: A Guide for Sufferers and Professionals*, Croom Helm, London.

Steuer, J., Bank, L. and Olsen, E.J. (1980) Depression, physical health and somatic complaints in the elderly: a study of the Zung Self-rating Depression Scale, *J. Gerontol.*, 35, 683–688.

Stuss, D. and Broughton, R. (1978) Extreme short sleep: personality profiles and a case study of sleep requirement, *Waking & Sleeping*, 2, 101–105.

Svanborg, A. (1985) The Gothenburg Longitudinal Study of 70-year-olds: clinical reference values in the elderly, in Bergener, M., Ermini, M. and Stehelin, H.B. (eds) *Thresholds in Aging.* pp. 231–239, Academic Press, London.

Turner, S.M., Jacob, R.G and Morrison, R. (1984) Somatoform and factitious disorders, in Adams, H.E. and Sutker, P.B. (eds) *Comprehensive Handbook of Psychopathology*, pp. 307–345, Plenum press, New York.

Walton, A. (1929) Rejuvenation: the work of Steinach and Voronoff, *Eugenics Rev.*, 20, 253–257.

Wattis, J. (1984) Is the patient confused or demented? *Geriatrics for G.P.s*, October.

Wells, C.E. (1979) Pseudodementia, *AM. J. Psychiat.*, 36, 895–900.

World Health Organization (1982) *Epidemiological Studies on Social and Medical Conditions of the Elderly, No. 62.* WHO, Copenhagen.

Young, M., Benjamin, B. and Wallis, G. (1963) Mortality of widowers, *The Lancet*, 2, 454.

Zarit, S.H. (1980) *Aging and Mental Disorders*, Macmillan Publishing Co., New York.

# 9

# Looking ahead to the twenty-first century

## THE CHANGING POPULATION STRUCTURE

Much of the matter of this book has been concerned with the fact that the age structure of Britain has radically altered during the twentieth century, and that this naturally has a significant effect on how older people are perceived in society, and how they perceive themselves, a factor that is relevant to their emotional well-being. This is not a phenomenon which is confined to the West and the most developed countries, but is world-wide. The increase in the number of people in the later decades of life has two main causes, as pointed out by Laslett (1989). First, the progress of medical science and general public health measures has caused people to live longer; second, the deliberate restriction of the size of families by methods of birth control means that there are proportionately fewer people in the younger age cohorts to replace those who are now aged. In Britain the records indicate that birth control began to be used to a significant degree in the 1870s in middle-class families, and the practice has spread to all classes in the present century, so that we are now a comparatively old community.

Few people have grasped the magnitude of the changes that will come in the twenty-first century. Malcolm Johnson, attempting to predict the problems of ageing in the next century, writes:

> At a recent international conference, I presented some simple figures about changing demographic patterns and mentioned that the number of people in Britain over 85 would grow from 560,000 now to over 1 million by the year 2000. But what really grabbed the attention of the media was a mere footnote

**Table 9.1** Projected population in three age groups for the 21st century (Great Britain). Figures in thousands. Percentages of total population shown

| AGE | 1987 | % | 2001 | % | 2016 | % | 2031 | % | 2046 | % | 2057 | % |
|---|---|---|---|---|---|---|---|---|---|---|---|---|
| **60–69** | | | | | | | | | | | | |
| Men | 2,620 | 4.7 | 2,502 | 4.3 | 3,154 | 5.4 | 3,710 | 6.2 | 2,910 | 5.0 | 3,362 | 5.8 |
| Women | 2,981 | 5.4 | 2,700 | 4.7 | 3,433 | 5.8 | 3,933 | 6.6 | 3,045 | 5.2 | 3,468 | 6.0 |
| Total | 5,601 | 10.1 | 5,202 | 9.0 | 6,587 | 11.2 | 7,643 | 12.8 | 5,955 | 10.2 | 6,830 | 11.9 |
| **70–79** | | | | | | | | | | | | |
| Men | 1,643 | 3.0 | 1,779 | 3.1 | 1,938 | 3.3 | 2,327 | 3.9 | 2,366 | 4.0 | 2,150 | 3.7 |
| Women | 2,404 | 4.3 | 2,320 | 4.0 | 2,384 | 4.1 | 2,851 | 4.8 | 2,841 | 4.9 | 2,557 | 4.4 |
| Total | 4,047 | 7.3 | 4,099 | 7.2 | 4,322 | 7.4 | 5,178 | 8.7 | 5,207 | 8.9 | 4,707 | 8.1 |
| **80+** | | | | | | | | | | | | |
| Men | 552 | 1.0 | 779 | 1.4 | 927 | 1.6 | 1,208 | 2.0 | 1,436 | 2.4 | 1,282 | 2.2 |
| Women | 1,338 | 2.4 | 1,651 | 2.8 | 1,668 | 2.8 | 2,036 | 3.4 | 2,386 | 4.1 | 2,150 | 3.7 |
| Total | 1,890 | 3.4 | 2,430 | 4.2 | 2,595 | 4.4 | 3,244 | 5.4 | 3,822 | 6.5 | 3,432 | 5.9 |
| **Grand Total for Age 60+** | 11,538 | 20.8 | 11,731 | 20.4 | 13,504 | 23.0 | 16,065 | 26.9 | 14,984 | 25.6 | 14,969 | 25.9 |

Source: Office of Population Censuses and Surveys (1987) *Population Projections by the Government Actuary PP2. No. 16.* HMSO, London.

that some biologists believe that small numbers of people will survive to the age of 130 by the middle of the next century. Radio, television and newspapers around the world found this relatively uncontroversial aside worthy of attention (Johnson, 1989, p. 62).

The fact that there may be some 130-year-olds around is not really of much significance; more importantly, we have to consider the huge increase in the number of those who are now considered to be the 'old old' (Neugarten, 1978). Will this label be shifted up another decade?

The figures for the future of the numbers in the elderly population in Great Britain, as computed by the Governmant Actuary (OPCS, 1987) are shown in Table 9.1.

Two trends may be noted in Table 9.1. First, while the numbers of all those over the age of 60 are expected to rise over the next half-century, the increase will be most marked in the cohort over the age of 80. This section includes those who are the frailest and in most need of medical and social services. How far improvements in public health, and in techniques for treating the disabilities of old age will improve, remains to be seen. The second trend to be noted is that although the numerical ratio of men to women in the later ages is expected to become less uneven as time goes on, the deficit of older men will continue.

All such projections for the future in the modern world in which so many technological and social changes are taking place are necessarily somewhat speculative, but at least they provide some guidelines for planning.

### Will there be a growing tension between the young and the old?

Old people don't earn any money and have to be paid a pension. They frequently suffer ills of the flesh so that their crumbling bodies clog up family doctors' waiting rooms and occupy an absurdly high proportion of costly hospital beds. Their younger relatives have better things to do than act as unpaid servants to wrinklies no longer capable of looking after themselves. In short oldies are a damned nuisance all round, and their numbers are increasing at an alarming rate. . . . There have been suggestions that before too long the state will

213

have to impose a statutory age limit on the right to life. This could involve oldsters receiving on, say, their 75th birthday, a buff OHMS envelope instructing them to attend their local euthanasia depot on the following Wednesday at 2.30 in the afternoon (Gould, 1987).

This article continues in a light and jocular manner suggesting ways in which the older members of the population could be disposed of for the benefit of the young. It is accompanied by a humorous cartoon to make it clear that it is not to be taken too literally. However, such humour serves to wrap up discussion of an idea that certainly betrays a tension within society, and having been shocked out of our complacency about the inevitability of humane standards in the civilized countries of Europe by one holocaust in the present century, we need to consider that tension seriously. The idea of the changing age-structure leading to a conflict between the generations is by no means new. In his younger days, Peter Medawar (1946) referred to the fact that in forty years' time we would become the victims of at least a numerical 'tyranny of greybeards', but he added 'a matter that does not worry me personally since I rather hope to be among their number'. However, in a humorous manner he mentioned the possibility of killing people at the age of seventy being a real kindness to them.

These, and other, jocular references to a possible state-enforced euthanasia as a means of getting rid of the excess of older people who are perceived as an intolerable burden on the public purse in the future are referred to by Laslett who comments:

But someone not too far away from his seventy-fifth birthday may perhaps be forgiven for asking if anyone so much as ventured to refer in passing to a holocaust of all black people in conversation with such persons as Medawar and Gould, let alone print and publish remarks to this effect. Nevertheless, we should not take sentiments such as these to be deliberately or realistically intended (Laslett, 1989, p. 99).

In the USA there is a small but vociferous body of opinion that complains that older people are being far too well treated, and are responsible for an unwarrantedly large share of the public purse, at the expense of the young. This viewpoint finds expression in such bodies as Americans for Generational Equity (AGE) as described by Minkler (1986). This source of inter-generational tension is particularly acute in the USA, because between the years 1946 and 1964 there was a huge 'baby boom' there, swelling the cohort of people who will reach the age of retirement in the early decades of the 21st century. This phenomenon has not been so apparent in the UK. Smith (1987) publishes a graphic figure showing that in 1955 each retired person had nearly nine individuals in the working population as 'supporters'. In the years 1975–2000 this drops to 3.5 'supporters', and by 2030 there are only two working people for every retired individual. The organization AGE protests that the older section of the population should not look to the public purse for support, but should be dependent on their own resources. This implies that everyone, knowing what future to expect, should contribute to private insurance schemes, or face a very impoverished old age.

This economically motivated form of ageism has not yet found any expression in an organized form in Britain, but some writers such as Johnson (1989) suggest that it is a possible development. We may examine the question by taking the projected figures of the Government Actuary as set out in Table 9.2.

In this table, the future point at which it is estimated that there will be the greatest percentage of older people in the population (as shown in Table 9.1) has been chosen for comparison with the present year, (1991). The 'working population', that is, those between the ages of 16 and retirement, may be seen to be 61.4% who are notionally supporting the remaining 38.6%, the larger

**Table 9.2** Comparison between the 'dependent' and the 'working' population (Great Britain). Figures in thousands. Percentages of total population shown

|  | 1991 | % | 2031 | % |
|---|---|---|---|---|
| Children below 16 years | 11,336 | 20.2 | 11,854 | 19.9 |
| Adults now retired (males 65+; females 60+) | 10,291 | 18.4 | 14,166 | 23.8 |
| Total dependants | 21,627 | 38.6 | 26,020 | 43.7 |
| Working population (Age 16 to retirement) | 34,360 | 61.4 | 33,592 | 56.3 |

Source: Office of Population Censuses and Surveys (1987) *Population Projections by the Government Actuary PP2. No. 16*, HMSO, London.

portion of which (20.2%) are children. In the year 2031 the 'working population' will be reduced to 56.3%, and they will be notionally responsible for the remaining 43.7%. Note that in the future the relative magnitudes of the percentages of children and retired people will be reversed.

All sorts of caveats must be observed in looking at these figures. It is highly unlikely that the present ages of retirement for men and women will be retained. It is more probable that people in their sixties in the year 2031, who were born in the 1970s, will be much fitter for their age than older people are today, and most of them will be part of the working population. Many people in their seventies and older may also be actively working. When we use the term 'the working population' we imply people who are actually productive in terms of goods and services, but many older people are owners of capital invested here and abroad, and are thus continuing to contribute to the productive process in terms of modern economics.

It is unlikely, therefore, that ageist conflict will develop in Britain along the lines suggested by the American organizers of AGE. Conflict between the generations on economic lines will doubtless continue, as discussed in Chapter 5, some younger people resenting their more affluent elders beginning to spend their money on themselves in enriching their lives, rather than living more parsimoniously and hoarding their money for their inheritors. Whether the larger number of people in the very oldest of the age cohorts who will continue to remain alive will be demanding a very much greater expenditure on health and social services, remains to be seen. According to the interesting model proposed by Fries (1980) that was discussed in Chapter 3, increased *efficiency* in medical and social care will mean that *less* should need to be spent in the future. It is projected that the 'survival curve' will become even more 'rectangular'; that is, the very old will maintain their health and fitness up to a certain point, and then go into a rapid and irreversible decline leading to their death.

## THE QUESTION OF AGEIST DISCRIMINATION

Forty years ago, legislation and social policies in Britain were modified to take account of the needs of 'the old'. The famous

Beveridge Report (Beveridge, 1942) had a special section devoted to 'The Problem of Age', which has been very influential in the post-war era, in affecting attitudes and policies concerning a growing section of the population who have reached certain ages held to be significant milestones. How far this now rather ramshackle structure of social security will last into the next century needs to be examined.

Who are 'the old'? We examined this question in Chapter 3 and it was apparent that no satisfactory answer could be found. Researches such as that of Ward (1984) in the USA, and the Gallup Poll in Britain (Sidhartha Films, 1984), that attempted to find out who regarded themselves as 'young', 'middle-aged', and 'old or elderly' produced no clear answer, for such appellations do not coincide at all closely with chronological age. The fact is that 'the old' is an unreal fiction; there is no such group, and if we pick arbitrarily on certain ages as milestones, then those who have lived beyond that age are by no means a homogeneous collection of people. Later, we shall examine the effects of choosing certain ages as milestones when enacting legislation and advising on social policies.

Because of the skewing of the age structure of the population towards the later years, we have become conscious of that form of bias and discrimination known as 'ageism', comparable to the prejudices of 'sexism' and 'racism' of which we have become more conscious in recent years. According to Marshall (1990) there has been a significant change for the better in public attitudes towards older people since about 1985; perhaps this progressive change will continue into the next century, but, as discussed earlier, it is by no means certain how far economic conditions may promote hostility to that part of the population who are living off pensions and require more medical care than younger people. It may be remarked that while we have laws against unfair discrimination that stems from sexism and racism, we have no laws against ageism.

It is necessary to consider how society is likely to change in the next century in response to the consciousness of ageist prejudice in our midst. Ageism has always been there but it has not been noticed until the late twentieth century, just as sexism was always there, but it was passively accepted by the great bulk of both men and women, until two world wars, among other historical factors, changed the status of women in our society. Here we have an interesting difference; men will never become women, and hence they will never be those who suffer directly from the worst effects of sexist prejudice; but everyone will eventually become old (unless they die young) so as the age structure of the population changes, more and more people will be forced to realize just which side of the fence they are on as regards ageist prejudice.

As well as the important changes brought about by the altered age structure of the population, there have been radical changes in public attitudes towards sexuality, and the emerging recognition that it is an important and valuable aspect of human life at all ages. What has sometimes been referred to as 'the sexual revolution' (London, 1978) occurred in the 1960s, and it has found official endorsement by the Western nations, as shown in the recommendations of the World Health Organization on human sexual education and freedom of expression (WHO, 1975) that have been quoted in Chapter 7.

### Older people as gaolers of 'the old'

It may be pointed out that just as a few women, deliberately or unthinkingly, appear to support some of the more extreme institutions of anti-feminist sexism, so certain older people appear to support the bastions upon which ageist prejudice depend. The organization Age Concern England sent out a questionnaire to several groups of people actively concerned with campaigning for adequate rights for older people. Such people might be expected to hold the most progressive attitudes to the issues that affect people in later life. The groups included their Retirement Forum, their National Organisations Forum, and its Age Concern Groups Forum. The results of this survery provide some surprises (Age Concern England, 1989). On the question concerning whether there should be age limits on the appointment to, and retirement from, statutory bodies, although some respondents answered that fitness for the job should be the criterion, others qualified their answers by such reservations as 'Provided that the member is still able to grasp and contribute to meetings', and similar caveats. Eric Midwinter comments on such caveats:

> Why add them, with their evocation of the doddering loon, slumped, with listless ear-trumpet, over the board table? Should not that proviso apply to *anybody* serving on *any*

committee? Is not the question more one of how we select and appoint committees in the first place? And these were positive ones and, remember, they come from within the 'old age' field itself where, incidentally, two groups reported that they had retirement ages for their own committees (Midwinter, 1990, p. 101).

Midwinter goes on to quote answers from representatives of elderly people who thought that age should be an *automatic* disqualifier for the holding of responsible office, such as 'Capability should be the main criteria (*sic*), but 70 years of age should be the limit.' A number of respondents cited the age of 70 as the upper age limit, and Midwinter comments that, 'While everyone else goes about believing 60 or 65 to be the correct retirement age, those who pride themselves on being positive about age have lifted the chronological sights to 70.' It seems then, that many of the more progressive older people who concern themselves with the plight of their elderly age-mates cannot re-adjust their values to the extent of questioning the ageist assumptions of the society in which they grew up. It is as if some women on boards and committees would not exclude all persons of the female sex from membership – only those who appeared *very* feminine, and some black members would not exclude all coloured people – only those who were *very* black!

In looking to the future, we must not expect the people who will be elderly in the twenty-first century to have the same attitudes as older people today. Some very interesting data on the attitudes of older people to important issues affecting those of their own generation are given by Clark (1989). He gives details of the seminars he was running as an activity of one of the larger branches of the University of the Third Age, over four years. This was in a relatively affluent area, and those attending the seminars were almost entirely from middle-class backgrounds, and about 85% of them were women. The title of the seminars was 'Living in the Third Age', and they were run as free discussion groups, there being no set syllabus, the group choosing to discuss whatever topics were of interest to them. An Appendix to the article lists the various topics that formed the basis of the discussions, and many of them concerned the sort of matters that have been dealt with in this book. However, it may be noted that the topics of re-marriage in later life and sexuality seem to have been largely ignored, although many of those attending were widowed or divorced. The following gives a sample of the attitudes expressed in the group:

> We sometimes discussed things that it was not appropriate for us to do. . . . It was certainly clear that we should not be irritable, cantankerous or drunken in public and we had the impression that sexual activity or interest on our parts was usually regarded with dismay when it was brought to the attention of the younger generation (Clark, 1989, p. 36).

This is a commentary on the younger generation as perceived by these older people, but it should be noted that they class even sexual *interest* with the unseemliness of public drunkenness. In the Victorian era much of the sexual behaviour and interest of young people had to be concealed from the censorial eyes of the older generation, but now it seems that such activity and interest among older people needs to be surreptitious, and concealed from the censorial eyes of the young – at least in the view of these people! As long as they hold this view, and behave accordingly, so will one of the powerful bastions of ageism be maintained.

Because people tend to behave and react according to the formative influences and education that they received when young, older people in our society have been slow to respond to the great changes in attitude towards sexuality that are now manifest, and are approved of by the World Health Organization recommendation referred to earlier. They still seem to feel as though there were Victorian parents, nannies and schoolteachers looking over their shoulders. Most of these people in the University of the Third Age were young adults during the war years or before, but looking to the future, it must be remembered that those who will be over 60 in the first decade of the twenty-first century were young adults during the 'swinging sixties'. Whatever their current attitudes are to 'the old', such people who are now middle-aged are unlikely to accept a restricted life when they themselves are old, and we may see very different patterns of living emerging among the older generations. The minority who are now campaigning on a number of fronts for full recognition of the rights of older people are preparing the way for the rising generations.

## Discrimination fair and unfair

We must consider how far ageist discrimination will persist into the next century. There is a danger that when people declare themselves against some form of discrimination, they forget that what they really mean is unfair and inappropriate discrimination. Some forms of age discrimination are obviously appropriate and necessary. We do not approve of young teenagers driving cars on the public roads. We recognize that they have not yet developed the requisite degree of judgement to engage in such a potentially dangerous activity, hence there is a minimum age limit for the granting of driving licenses. It may be argued that some children of the age of fourteen would be as competent and responsible car-drivers as most of those aged 18, and this is certainly true, but the potential danger is too great for the risk to be taken of granting driving licenses to everyone at the age of 14.

The same difficult questions apply when considering the upper ranges of the age spectrum. Midwinter (1990) has questioned the use of an upper age bar in a number of fields – appointment to, and retirement from, the judiciary, jury service, membership of statuary bodies, voluntary committees, the ambulance service, and various similar posts where both adequate competence and sound judgement are needed. He refers to the Department of Health's stipulation regarding the appointment of people to the District Health Authorities:

> it is important to make appointments only where it is likely that prospective members will have the health and vigour to make an effective contribution throughout their term of office. Appointment or re-appointment over the age of 65 should be regarded as exceptional and should only be offered if equally suitable younger candidates are not available (Department of Health, 1981).

The important consideration is, of course, what checks there are on the all-round fitness of members to fulfil their duties, whether they are under or over the age of 65, which is a pretty meaningless milestone anyway. The danger lies in people occupying positions of power where their general performance is not subject to much scrutiny from colleagues or those they serve. This is particularly critical for members of the judiciary. The Lord Chancellor's Department has stipulated that in the selection of magistrates, 'candidates must be below the age of 60 and preference is normally given to those under 50'. Here we come upon two possible reasons for diminishing fitness with ageing; ceasing to be properly in touch with the mores of the younger generations, and actual subtle but relevant deterioration of judgement due to the disease processes that affect the brain in a minority of people in later life. Lay magistrates on the juvenile panel are expected to retire at age 65, and other magistrates at age 70, but whether those over 65 are really less competent to deal with juveniles is sheer speculation based on ageist assumptions that are probably unsound. However, the danger of a subtle deterioration of judgement in some cases, due to the onset of brain disease, is a real risk that must be faced. We discussed in Chapter 8 how diseases of the Alzheimer type are insidious in their onset, and affect both memory and judgement. Some figures were given as to the known incidence of such disease in older age groups: Bennet (1989) suggests that about one in ten of the population over the age of 65 have some form of dementia, and one in five of those over 85, and Johnson (1989) states that 'dementia of the Alzheimer type will affect between 5% and 15% of people over 75.' Even if this is an over-estimate, as Bennet admits, it is pretty certain that in days gone by when many serving judges were in their eighties, some of them were in the early stages of deterioration due to diseases of the Alzheimer type, and some of the extraordinary homilies and sentences they handed out were probably due to a pathological deterioration of judgement. Such judges could be retired by the Lord Chancellor, but only after some harm had been done, and extra work incurred by the appeal courts. A few others in their 50s are no doubt the victims of the early stages of Alzheimer-type diseases, but short of having judges and magistrates subjected to periodic medical and psychological testing, there is not much we can do about it. It seems a reasonable compromise, therefore, to retire judges before their 80s, even though some perfectly competent individuals will have their careers terminated prematurely.

The above is an extreme example of the appropriateness of some forms of age discrimination in later life, just as is the restriction of the granting of driving licenses to those who are beyond their early teens. In looking forward to the twenty-first century, therefore, we should not react to the unfair ageism of the present century by throwing overboard all acknowledgement of the fact that age is indeed a meaningful parameter, but learn to use discrimination fairly and appropriately. Failure to recognize the significant aspects of age results in many emotional maladjustments and consequent unhappiness and ill-health. In Chapters 6 and 7 it was pointed out that many of the emotional problems some men encounter in later life are due to their failure to recognize and allow for the normal and inevitable physiological changes that take place in their sexual capacity with ageing. They need not become 'asexual', but they must learn how to express their sexuality in somewhat different ways.

The example of Alzheimer type degenerative brain conditions, much more common in later life, creating discriminatory practices that are perhaps justifiable, highlights the need for biomedical research aimed to eradicate such diseases. Society must decide how much priority is to be accorded to competing research aimed at improving the lot of different sections of the population. When people in the older section of the population become even more numerous, and, it is to be hoped, more vocal, it is natural that priorities will change.

## SOCIAL SECURITY IN THE FUTURE

In Chapter 3 it was pointed out that some time ago commercial interests realized that there was a good deal of money to be made by appealing to those of the retired generation who were relatively affluent. New magazines have appeared appealing to older people, and advertising all sorts of goods and services attractive to them. Previously, in later life people had been wont to save their money for the sake of their children who would inherit it, but this pattern has been breaking down and the 'new old' are being encouraged to spend their money on living life to the full. A high rate of inflation encourages such patterns of free spending. This relatively affluent section of the older population has been humorously referred to as the 'Woopies' (Well Off Older People) and the 'Jollies' (Jet-setting Oldies with Lots of Loot), but the conspicuous nature of the free-spending section of the older population should not blind us to the more general standard of living for retired people at present.

Before considering how Social Security will develop in the twenty-first century, we must consider the position as it is now in the 1990s. The plain fact is that most people over pensionable age are living in considerably straightened circumstances. In the Welfare State, poverty is still with us, and most poor people are poor because they are elderly. Taking the figures of the Department of Social Security (DSS, 1989) which are for very recent years, about a million pensioners have been living on incomes below the poverty line of the Supplementary Benefit. We may ask why, in a formal democracy such as we have in Britain, so many older people put up with living out the rest of their lives in poverty? Their poverty is reflected in all sorts of measures of deprivation as shown in such studies as that of Mack and Lansley (1985): they are inadequately housed, they lack proper heating in cold weather, their diet is poor and they show a lack of consumer durables. Various forms of disability are more common in later life among poorer people, and we have already seen how the numbers in the most vulnerable elderly group will greatly increase in the coming century. Being somewhat disabled costs money. Evidence published by the Office of Population Censuses and Surveys (Martin et al., 1988) indicated that pensioners with minor disabilities needed to pay an extra £5.70 per week, and those with severe disabilities spent an extra £10.50 a week. This was in 1985, but Thompson et al. (1988) have claimed that these figures greatly underestimate the true extent to which disability among pensioners involves extra expenditure.

Britain is not a particularly poor country among others of the European community, yet pensioners here are considerably worse off. Chapman (1990) has shown that among nine member countries of the EEC Britain came second to last in the standard of living of pensioners. The purchasing power of a single person's pension in Britain is only 50% of that of the Dutch pensioner, 60% of the West German pensioner, and less than 75% of the French. Whatever may be the cause of these differences between the European countries, the attitude of the British towards their own poverty is reflected in the fact that, according to the Department of Social Security, in 1985 900,000 people failed to claim the benefits to which they were entitled, and this applied particularly to Supplementary Benefit – 79% of elderly people who were entitled to it failed to claim it (DSS, 1989). Is this due to irrational pride, to apathetic acceptance of poverty, or mainly to a strong revulsion from having any truck with bureaucracy? Evandrou and Falkingham (1989) suggest that the failure of many frail older people to ask for the benefits they are entitled to is because they fail to realize that what they suffer from is due to definable and perhaps remediable forms of disability, and not the inevitable concomitants of old age. The age cohorts who will be pensioners in the coming century will have had a different social history, and be better educated, so they are less likely to be prepared to tolerate the continuance of the conditions that exist today. It is possible that if in the next century Britain becomes much more closely tied in as an economic unit within the European community, the standard of living of the older section of the population will improve, and become more like that of our European neighbours.

Some social scientists such as Walker (1990) argue strongly that the whole system of the retirement pensions that was built into the social security scheme following the Beveridge Report has been responsible for a pernicious form of age discrimination. Superficially it saves the Treasury money, but in fact it helps to build up a large pool of ill-health and disability which are a drain on the health services both now and for the future. If the voice of the growing number of older citizens is heard in the next century, what progressive amendments to the present system can we hope to see? One pressing area that calls for reform concerns those who have some significant disability. At present, their full needs are not acknowledged and, by a strange anomaly, they are denied the benefits that are available to younger people who are disabled, since people are regarded as being unfit for work *either* by reason of disability, *or* by reason of age. In the future we may hope to see a comprehensive disability scheme which is unrelated to age. This, of course, should be flexible enough to cover all eventualities. A person who cannot work, say, by reason of impaired vision, will need an extra income in later life if mobility becomes hampered by severe arthritis, and the pension should be as of right and not affected thereby.

People have grown up to expect to be poorer in later life and to have to stint themselves a little as they get older, but there is no reason why this should be if there were a real system of social welfare. Why should not everybody expect a greater degree of affluence in later life and this be planned for by a system of social security very different from that envisaged by Beveridge? Obviously if such changes come about in the next century ample provision must be made for younger adults who have the responsibility for rearing families, but already the principle of family allowances is acknowledged.

No blue-print for a future incomes policy is being attempted here, but if one is seriously to consider the general well-being of older people in the altered society of the future their material security must be considered, and new perspectives must be attempted. The spectre of the Poor Law, tempered by benificent private charity, still haunts the people who were born in the early decades of this century. It is patronizing to allow older persons various 'concessions'. For instance, they are allowed to travel at a lower rate on public transport – provided they travel at the correct time of day – but it would be more in keeping with their dignity and conception of their value as citizens, if they had a decent income and hence could afford to pay the same as all other adults. The spirit of the much-parodied Victorian poem 'Twas Christmas Day in the Workhouse' still finds expression in the £10 tip that is given to pensioners at Christmas time.

## MEDICAL ASPECTS OF AGEING IN THE FUTURE

In the twentieth century the outstanding developments in medicine, that have partly been responsible for changing age structure, concerned the conquest of most of the parasitic and infectious diseases, and preventive measures such as innoculation have almost eliminated many of such conditions. Diphtheria, poliomyelitis, syphilis, and tuberculosis, to mention but a few of them, no longer account for the premature death of a significant part of the population as in earlier times. In Chapter 8, the chief causes of illness and death in the later decades of life were discussed, and it was pointed out that there is a strong connection between the sort of life-style that older people achieve, their general contentment and emotional well-being, and their medical status and longevity. The view that there are 'two nations' among the elderly population is supported by the fact that those of the professional and managerial class enjoying a relatively affluent life-style live considerably longer than people in the unskilled working class. The ten years' difference in life expectancy of these two groups is not, of course, produced solely by contrasting life-styles after retirement, but poverty in later life and all that goes with it exacerbates the ills that have been accruing during many years of sub-optimal health.

How people will age in the twenty-first century is not, there-fore, solely the responsibility of medical and other health-care professionals; economic, social and political factors will deter-mine the framework within which the health-care services can work. But with regard to more direct medical responsibility in the future we may quote Lord Butterfield, 'it would not be a bad thing if a major objective for medicine in the next century was the protection and maintenance of brain function!' (Butterfield 1989, p. 12). Here the relative affluence or poverty of older people has little relation to the development of degenerative diseases of the Alzheimer type, but where organic brain deterio-ration is of the multi-infarct type, the life-style and general health of older people is certainly relevant. Lord Butterfield goes on to point out that:

> What leads to serious deterioration of brain function seems to be the effects of intercurrent illnesses and operations which interfere with the brain's nutrition. This can occur during periods of severe respiratory infections or due to trouble with the brain arteries running through the bones of the neck, or due to little strokes from very small clots getting swept up into the brain, or little blocks in the smaller arteries needed to nourish the brain. So there is a school of medical thought which tries to preserve the brain by paying special attention to elderly people when they get ill (Butterfield, 1989, p. 14).

While doctors, nurses and other health-care professionals can apply all their skills in looking after older people when they run the risk of incurring vascular infarcts and subsequent brain deterioration through periods of sickness, basically it comes back to the question of individuals having sufficient enjoyment of life, and hence the will to look after themselves even in adverse economic circumstances. By striving to preserve themselves in optimal health, they have a much better chance of retaining their intellectual functions. In effect, a better-educated public in the future should become more collaborators with health-care pro-fessionals in a joint effort to preserve health and well-being, rather than just being the passive recipients of services, as has been the case too often in the past.

Many people in the oldest age cohorts today still retain attitudes of suspicion towards health-care workers. This is understandable, for social workers are modern representatives of the relieving officers of the Poor Law, and doctors used to be feared as possible agents whereby dreaded surgical operations were initiated. Boxes of pills and bottles of nasty-tasting coloured water were what most patients had to depend on for most of their ills, before the advent of effective drugs and treatments. We have now entered a totally new era of medicine in which professionals no longer need to hide their ignorance of many health-care matters by the assumption of a mask of all-knowing inscrutability, but actually seek to educate the public in the technicalities of the maintenance of health as far as possible. Some modern general practitioners provide in their waiting rooms a library of books on numerous aspects of health-care, and encourage patients to read, and become knowledgeable about various medical conditions. Such an approach would have been strongly disapproved of by many doctors of the old school. Equipped with such information, their patients stand the best chance of avoiding becoming ill and disabled. The dissemination of reliable medical knowledge also serves to prevent patients from becoming the victims of much of the present-day quackery that presents itself in the guise of 'alternative medicine', and appeals to people who have very little education in matters of health-care. How far this trend can be developed in the future remains to be seen.

Here we have a paradox: the medical profession, along with other health-care professions, is changing in a progressive direction as regards older people, but not all younger doctors are more enlightened in their attitudes than older ones. According to Lehr (1987), 'the older the doctor or the nurse, the more effectively they foster self-reliant, independent behaviour in the elderly patient. Younger doctors and nurses, on the other hand, tend to encourage dependent behaviour and passivity on the part of their patients' (pp. 114–115). This is a subject about which it is difficult to be too definite and make generalizations. The subject was discussed in Chapter 4 concerning the training of professionals, and because of the rising number of older people, professionals of the future will have to become more familiar with key issues in gerontology and geriatric medicine. These were once very minor specialisms, but obviously they will become increasingly important.

## MARRIAGE AND SEXUALITY IN THE TWENTY-FIRST CENTURY

If we are to consider what forms of marriage and expression of sexuality in later life may develop in the twenty-first century, it is necessary to consider what likely or possible changes may take place in these matters for the whole community. We have already seen how the conventional institution of monogamous marriage that is ideally life-long has changed during the latter part of the current century. About one in three marriages now ends in divorce, but the institution is still maintained because the great majority of divorced people re-marry. Most people still appear to live in monogamous marriages, although there is now a greater tolerance for extra-marital affairs. It is very difficult to get reliable data on this matter, but what appears to have changed is that where previously husbands' extramarital behaviour was often tolerated, now more wives have taken this freedom for themselves, without necessarily breaking the marriage. It may be said that whereas the marriage contract used to be life-long for the overwhelming majority of people, now there is a greater tendency for there to be serial marriages.

These changes in the institution of marriage have reflected the great modifications of sexual mores that have taken place in the post-war era. Thus if we compare the findings of Kinsey *et al.* (1948; 1953) with those of Hunt (1974) we find that some very significant developments in sexual practices have taken place over a quarter of a century. Kinsey and his colleagues found that over 25% of unmarried males had not had sexual intercourse by the age of 25 years, but Hunt found that the number of male virgins of that age was only 3%. For unmarried females, Kinsey found that about 70% were virgin up to the age of 25, but in Hunt's survey only about 30% had not experienced intercourse by that age. Among females who had married by the age of 25, Kinsey found that about 45% had engaged in pre-marital intercourse, whereas Hunt found the percentage to be 81%.

This significant change was confirmed by a slightly later study involving 100,000 women readers of the magazine *Redbook*. Levin and Levin (1975) found that 90% of all married respondents to a readership survey under the age of 25 had had pre-marital intercourse, and there was a steady increase in the rate for those married after 1964. Extramarital affairs were admitted to by

30% of these women, and such affairs were positively related to the age at which these women had started pre-marital sex. In Kinsey's study, only 9% of all wives (whatever their age) admitted to having extra-marital affairs.

But perhaps the most significant change that has been occurring is that the double standard in sexual mores appears to have been crumbling, for Hunt's research showed that while there had been a moderate increase over the years in the number of men under 25 having extra-marital sex, there had been a large increase among women of that age.

These data about the sexual behaviour of younger people and its relation to marriage are, of course, relevant to the coming years when such people will be elderly. Throughout this book there has been a stress on how early influences on patterns of behaviour condition the attitudes manifest when people are older. In later life, marriages are broken not only by divorce and separation, but by bereavement, and hence the possibility of re-marriage arises, constrained as it is by the growing numerical disparity between the sexes. While many older people may contentedly pursue their sex-lives without bothering to obtain any sort of legal and social sanction, some do, in fact, feel the need for an official recognition of their unions. The religious view of marriage expressed in Christian churches has gradually developed from an essentially negative attitude to the sexual aspect of it, to a positive recognition of its value. The Church used to justify the practice of sexual intercourse within marriage because of the need for procreation, and for the avoidance of the greater sin of fornication, but more recently the potential of sex for expressing and consolidating interpersonal love has become recognized, as it always has been in the Jewish and Muslim faiths, and in the other great world religions. However, in the past Christian belief has not always been inconsistent with forms of marriage very different from the officially approved type of monogamous union prevalent today, as in the history of the Mormon Church, and the Oneida Community whose leader, John Humphrey Noyes, regarded contemporary marriage as being inconsistent with the Bible, and inaugurated a strange form of sexual communism as described by Parker (1972). We may yet see new forms of marriage and sexual union developing in the next century in response to demographic and other changes.

## The male prophets for the future

Jessie Bernard (1982) discusses the future of marriage in terms of 'the male prophets' and 'the female prophets'. About the most interesting of the former is the science fiction writer Paul Anderson, who suggests that in the future people may go through three successive types of marital union: (i) a form designed to satisfy sexual urges; (ii) for procreative and child-rearing purposes; (iii) to secure mature companionship. Males would pass through these three types in succession, first beginning at about the age of 16 with an experienced woman older than themselves, and after about 10 years taking a teen-age wife for procreative purposes when they are in their late 20s. When the children of such a marriage were about six years old, they would be handed over to the state for rearing, and the man, then in his 40s, would contract a third form of marriage with a woman of similarly mature years to secure lasting companionship. In this scheme, women would go through the stages in the order of (ii), (i), (iii), that is, first beginning in their adolescence with a much older husband, to go through their period of procreation, and when this was completed in their 30s, forming a union that was, from their point of view, primarily for purposes of sexual enjoyment. Such a scheme should not be dismissed out of hand as bizarre, because anthropology and history have shown that very diverse forms of marriage have existed, and still exist, in various cultures at different times.

A great number of criticisms and objections to Paul Anderson's three-stage scheme for marriage may be advanced which need not be discussed here. As far as it concerns people in the later decades of life, it provides no answer to the difficulty that women far outnumber men to an increasing extent after the age of 60, and it is unlikely that this discrepancy will be resolved, at least in the first half of the twenty-first century. Victor Kassel (1975) has suggested a scheme designed to meet this difficulty. His proposal is that men over the age of 60 should be permitted to marry from two to five women in their own age-group at the same time, and he believes that a genuine 'family group', with perhaps some blood-relatives in the greatly extended family would develop in such a system. It would certainly enable a number of women to pool their material resources in their later years, and to ensure

231

a network of relationships which would sustain the more frail members as they age. But such an arrangement would entirely overlook one important fact. Polygyny for a younger man is feasible if he has the sexual capacity to satisfy several women, but as the sexual capacity of the male declines more rapidly in later life than that of the female, most men over the age of 60 would prove to be rather unsatisfactory husbands to their wives. In terms of sheer companionship and economic stability such an arrangement might have its advantages, yet what little we know about the subject indicates that men and women in our culture are no less jealous in later life than they are when young, and many women who have not grown up in a harem-oriented society might find such a marriage intolerable.

Having discussed the male prophets' schemes for the future of marriage, Jessie Bernard gives as her verdict:

There is something rather stale, unimaginative, unexciting and quite *déjà vu* about the array of possible options they offer us. We have heard it and seen it all before. . . . Many of the modern male prophets seem so hung up on their male biases that, try as they may, they keep coming up with the same old stuff. Nor have they come to terms with the spirited nature of the women they are going to have to live with whatever their form of marriage may take, women who do not have their biases and are far more in tune with the tenor of the times. The women prophets are zeroing on the crucial problems and coming up with far more interesting answers (Bernard, 1982, p. 209).

### The female prophets

Jessie Bernard goes on to discuss the female prophets, the most important of whom she finds among the young, avant-garde radical women of the 'Female of Women's Liberation Movement'. In her words, 'Such women no longer see marriage as the goal of every woman, and some even talk seriously of celibacy'. We may remark, in passing, that such a sentiment might be regarded as distinctly *déjà vu* by most feminists of the old school, and their male supporters such as Ibsen, Shaw, Wells, Russell, etc.!

When we come to examine the schemes of these radical feminist prophets for the future, we find that some would dispense with marriage altogether, and some, such as Kearon (1970) are self-confessed man-haters, and make their hatred quite explicit. A few of these young women envisage life-long celibacy, as some religious women have throughout the centuries, but according to Bernard, the great majority are neither 'anti-marriage' nor for 'non-marriage'.

Examining the proposals of the majority of the radical feminists who do not reject marriage we find very little that is constructive as far as they might affect women in later life who have a real problem. The chief demand of these younger women is a very reasonable one: that in marriage, men and women should have equal rights and respect one another, and that by building up networks of 'sisterhood', women should achieve a goal of 'personhood', and jointly resist any encroachment on their rights and dignity by sexist husbands. Viewed with hindsight from the 1990s, we may marvel a little at the degree of emotional rhetoric with which such a point of view was put forward in the 1970s. Unfortunately these younger radical feminists appear to be concerned only with the problems of those in their own generation, and do not consider that women in the later decades of life have special problems now, and moreover, that one day they themselves will be elderly and living in a society that is significantly different from that which they experience today. Barbara Macdonald, a feminist campaigner who is now in her 70s, describes how she has come to be rejected by the younger members of the women's movement because they assume that at her age she can no longer be regarded as a relevant and valuable 'sister' (Macdonald and Rich, 1985).

The feminist who has provided the most useful suggestion for a modification to the institution of marriage in the coming century is the late Margaret Mead (1966). She proposed that there should be two forms of marriage; one form should be sheerly contractual and carry no rights of inheritance. This would be particularly suitable for men and women in later life who wish to live together and have their union officially recognized, but do not wish to provoke the sort of family conflicts over the inheritance of property that were discussed in Chapter 5. Children of a former marriage might be happier if their mother or father formed such a union that did not in any way threaten

233

their right of inheritance. A marriage of this form could be contracted at any age, but if children resulted from the union, it would then be automatically converted into the conventional form of marriage which gives protection for children and puts legal obligations and responsibilities on both partners.

The lack of awareness and neglect of the problems of older people, both now and for the future, that is characteristic of the feminist movement that arose in the 1960s is manifest in Jessie Bernard's book. It is a book of substantial size, yet it devotes only just over one page to what is called 'geriatric marriage'. Here the term 'geriatric' is not being used correctly, for it properly refers to the medical treatment of illness in old age (*geras* = old age; *iatrikos* = healing), and has become rather a derogatory term implying that ageing is a form of sickness. In Bernard's book with the title of *The Future of Marriage*, this trivial reference to something that is becoming of increasing social importance, is perhaps surprising.

## The lesbian alternative

Quite a lot of attention has been paid to Jessie Bernard's book in this section because there are relatively few books that are devoted to discussing the future of the institution of marriage and the alternatives for the expression of love and achieving sexual fulfilment. Surprisingly, lesbianism is not mentioned at all, not for the 'man-haters', nor for those who would reject all sexual advances from men. Homosexual relations between women have never been criminal in this country and perhaps there has never been a time when there has been greater social tolerance for them in Britain. There is now quite a body of contemporary literature discussing lesbianism, much of it being written by feminists who regard it as a natural alternative for those who do not wish to be involved sexually with men. As there is a great shortage of available men in the later decades of life, it would seem that there is a reasonable case for single women forming lesbian associations with one another, even though they have been exclusively heterosexual in their younger years.

When many men are deprived of female company it is well known that they turn rather easily to homosexual behaviour, as in prisons, the navy, and other all-male communities. Although a similar phenomenon is to be observed among women, as in convents, boarding schools etc., the tendency is far less pronounced. The Kinsey studies, and all subsequent surveys of human sexuality, have shown a far greater prevalence of homosexual behaviour among men than among women. In the extensive survey of Brecher (1984) of the sexual behaviour of men and women over 50, 301 (13%) of the men admitted to having had homosexual relationships, but only 131 (8%) of the women admitted this. This survey also asked the question 'Have you ever felt sexually attracted to a person of your own gender?' Here, rather surprisingly, more women than men admitted to having felt homosexual attraction. Brecher seeks to explain these findings in terms of the very different upbringings that girls and boys experienced in the earlier part of this century when they were young, the girls having been subjected to stronger taboos about sex. It may be that in the next century, older men and women, having experienced more liberal treatment in childhood, and having lived in a society that is more tolerant of homosexual behaviour, will have attitudes that are more similar, and that single elderly women will be more prone to form lesbian relationships than they are now.

## REFERENCES

Age Concern England (1989) *Retirement Forum: Responses to Questionnaire* (unpublished), Age Concern, London.
Bennet, G. (1989) *Alzheimer's Disease and Other Confusional States*, McDonald Optima, London.
Bernard, J. (1982) *The Future of Marriage*, Yale University Press, New Haven.
Beveridge, W. (1942) *Social Insurance and Allied Services*, Cmd 6404, HMSO, London.
Brecher, E.M. (1984) *Love, Sex and Aging: A Consumer Union Report*, Little, Brown & Co, Boston.
Butterfield, J. (1989), Medicine into the 21st century, in Futerman, V. (ed.) *Into the 21st Century*, pp. 11–16, University of the Third Age in Cambridge.
Chapman, K. (1990) Looking around Europe, *Eurolink Age Bulletin*, March.
Clark, D.H. (1989) Living in the third age: a report on U3A discussion groups 1984–1988, in Futerman, V. (ed.) *Into the 21st Century*, pp. 30–39, University of the Third Age in Cambridge.
Department of Health (1981) *Circular H.C. 15*, HMSO, London.

Department of Social Security (1989) *Supplementary Benefit Take-up 1985/86: Technical Note*, DSS, London.

Evandrou, M. and Falkingham, J. (1989) Benefit discrimination, *Community Care*, 25th May.

Fries, J.F. (1980) Ageing, natural death and the compression of morbidity, *New Eng. J. Med.*, 303, 130–135.

Gould, D. (1987) Death by decree, *New Scientist*, 114 (1560), 65.

Hunt, M.M. (1974) *Sexual Behavior in the 1970s*, Dell Publishing Co, New York.

Johnson, M. (1989) Ageing in the 21st Century, in Futerman, V. (ed.) *Into the 21st Century*, pp. 61–71, University of the Third Age in Cambridge.

Kassel, V. (1975) Polygyny after 60, in Kammeyer, K.C.W. (ed.) *Confronting the Issues*, pp. 113–120, Allyn & Bacon, Boston.

Kearon, P. (1970) Man-hating, in *Notes From the Second Year*, Women's Liberation. Cited by Bernard, J. (1982) *The Future of Marriage*, Yale University Press, New Haven.

Kinsey, A.C., Pomeroy, W.B. and Martin, C.E. (1948) *Sexual Behavior in the Human Male*, W.B. Saunders, Philadelphia.

Kinsey, A.C., Pomeroy, W.B., Martin, C.E. and Gebhard, P.H. (1953) *Sexual Behavior in the Human Female*, W.B. Saunders, Philadelphia.

Laslett, P. (1989) *A Fresh Map of Life*, Weidenfeld & Nicholson, London.

Lehr, U. (1987) The elderly patient in medical practice, in Meier-Page, W. (ed.) *The Elderly Patient in General Practice*, Karger, Basle.

Levin, R.J. and Levin, A. (1975) Sexual pleasure: the surprising preferences of 100,000 women, *Redbook*, September, 51–58.

London, P. (1978), Sexual behavior, in Reich, W.T. (ed.) *Encyclopedia of Bioethics*, pp. 1560–1568, The Free Press, New York.

Macdonald, B. and Rich, C. (1985), *Look Me in the Eye: Old Women, Ageing and Ageism*, The Women's Press, London.

Marshall, M. (1990) Proud to be old, in McEwan, E. (ed.) *Age: The Unrecognized Discrimination*, pp. 28–42, Age Concern, London.

Mack, J. and Lansley, S. (1985), *Poor Britain*, Allen & Unwin, London.

Martin, J., Meltzer, H. and Elliott, D. (1988) *The Prevalence of Disability Among Adults, Report 1*, HMSO, London.

Mead, M. (1966) Marriage in two steps, *Redbook*, July.

Medawar, P.B. (1946) *The Uniqueness of the Individual*, Constable, London.

Midwinter, E. (1990) Your country doesn't need you! Age discrimination and voluntary service, in McEwan, E. (ed.) *Age: The Unrecognized Discrimination*, pp. 97–106, Age Concern, London.

Minkler, M. (1986) 'Generational equity' and the new victim blaming: an emerging public policy issue, *Int. J. Health Services*, 16, 539–550.

Neugarten, B. (1978) Social implications of aging, in Reich, W.T. (ed.) *Encyclopedia of Bioethics*, pp. 54–58, The Free Press, New York.

Office of Population Censuses and Surveys (1987), *Population Projections by* the Government Actuary, PP2. No. 16, HMSO, London.

Parker, R.A. (1972) *A Yankee Saint: John Humphrey Noyes and the*

*Oneida Community*, The Porcupine Press, Philadelphia.

Sidhartha Films Ltd. (1974) *The Elderly*, Gallup Poll, London.

Smith, L. (1987), The war between the generations, *Fortune* July 20, 50–53.

Thompson, P., Buckle, J. and Lavery, M. (1988) *Not in the OPCS Survey*, Disability Income Group, London.

Walker, A. (1990) The benefits of old age? Discrimination and social security, in McEwan, E. (ed.) *Age: The Unrecognized Discrimination*, pp. 58–70, Age Concern, London.

Ward, R.A. (1984), *The Aging Experience*. New York: Harper & Row.

World Health Organization (1975) *Education and Treatment in Human Sexuality, Technical Report No. 572*, WHO, Geneva.

# Appendices

## APPENDIX A
## BOOKS SUITABLE FOR RECOMMENDATION TO OLDER CLIENTS AND PATIENTS

Bristow, P. (ed.) (1990) *Famous Ways to Grow Old*, Age Concern, London.
This is an edited collection of letters from older people who are well-known in various fields, giving their personal views on growing old. It provides inspiration for all of us meeting the challenges of ageing.

Brown, P. and Faulder, C. (1979) *Treat Yourself to Sex*, Penguin Books, Harmondsworth.
This is not written specifically for older people, but it contains much useful information and advice concerning personal and sexual relationships.

Butler R.N. and Lewis, M.I. (1988) *Love and Sex After 60*, revised edn, Harper & Row, New York.
This is about the best all-round guide to the various personal and sexual problems encountered in later life written by two eminent authorities in the field of gerontology and well-written for the lay public.

Cole, M. and Dryden, W. (1989) *Sex Problems: Your Questions Answered*, Macdonald & Co, London.
This is very simply written in a question-and-answer format. While not specifically concerned with older people, it is highly informative about a great variety of sexual matters, and provides information about where to go for help with minority problems. £4.99.

Comfort, A. (1990) *A Good Age*, Pan Books, London.
This book was first published in 1977, and has now been fully revised and appears in paperback. It is an excellent discussion of all the important social, emotional and physical problems that face people when ageing and is highly readable. It is to be recommended very highly. £5.95.

Greengross, W. and Greengross, S. (1989) *Living, Loving and Ageing*. Age Concern, London.
This has the advantage of being expressly concerned with older people, and is easily comprehensible by the less educated readers. Most of the book is about sexuality, and it deals briefly with other problems. £4.95.

Marriott, V. and Timblick, T. (1988) *Loneliness – How to Overcome It*, Age Concern, London.

The first author is an 'agony aunt', and the book contains letters she has received from people with problems of loneliness. It gives much useful advice about coping with such problems, and includes addresses of many self-help organizations. £3.95.

Masters, W.H., Johnson, V.E. and Kolodny (1986) *Sex and Human Loving*, Macmillan, London.

This is a very readable account of a great variety of expressions of love and sexuality, and is addressed to the more intelligent reading public. It is also a very useful reference book.

West, S. (1990) *Your Rights*, Age Concern, London.

This is a general guide to the State benefits that are available to older people.

Young, P. (1986) *At Home in a Home*, Age Concern, London.

When elderly people consider moving into a home they ask many questions about what it entails and what it will be like. This book sets out to answer such questions.

## APPENDIX B

## WHERE OLDER PEOPLE AND THEIR CARERS CAN BE REFERRED FOR HELP AND ADVICE

Alzheimer's Disease Society
158–160 Balham High Road
London SW12 9BN Tel. 071-675-6557

This society publishes a Newsletter, a number of factsheets, and gives guidance for people who are caring for patients suffering from the disease.

Amarant Trust
14 Lord North Street
London SW1P 3LD Tel. 071-401-3855

This trust is concerned with giving information about menopausal problems and hormone replacement therapy.

Arthritis Care
5 Grosvenor Crescent
London SW1X 7ER Tel-071-235-0902

Information and support is offered on the general problems of coping with arthritis, and it has some local branches.

Association to Aid the Sexual and Personal Relationships of People with a Disability (SPOD)
286 Camden Road
London N7 OBJ Tel. 071-607-8851

This is an advisory and counselling service for those who have some sexual problem due to a physical or mental disability. It gives information to health-care workers and to individual clients.

Association of Sexual and Marital Therapists
PO Box 62
Sheffield S10 3TL
> This is the association to which most qualified sex therapists belong. They have a list of approved therapists in all parts of the country which is available to professionals and to members of the public who should send a s.a.e. Its members work both privately and for the NHS.

Cancerlink
17 Brittania Street
London WC1X 9JN Tel. 071-833-2451
> This provides support for self-help groups in various parts of Britain, and gives information about all aspects of cancer.

Carers' National Association
29 Chilworth Mews
London W2 3RG Tel. 071-724-7776
> This is a charity which aims to develop support for those caring for elderly and handicapped people, and to bring their needs to the attention of policy-makers.

Chest, Heart and Stroke Association
Tavistock House North,
Tavistock Square,
London WC1H 9JH Tel. 071-387-3012
> This is concerned with health education, and offering counselling services and rehabilitation to victims of related disabilities.

Colostomy Welfare Group
38/39 Eccleston Square
London SW1V 1PB Tel. 071-828-5175
> Patients who have had a colostomy operation, and those caring for them, are offered advice, and practical help if necessary.

CRUSE Bereavement Care
126 Sheen Road
Richmond
Surrey TW9 1UR Tel. 081-940-4818
> Bereaved people are offered counselling and general supportive social services which are locally based.

Friend
274 Upper Street
London N1 2UA
also:
Box BM Friend
London WC1N 3XX Tel. 071-837-3337
> This organization offers help and information to both men and women who are homosexual.

Gay Men's Disabled Group
c/o Gay's The Word Bookshop

66 Marchmont Street
London WC1N 1AB Tel-071-278-7654

> This group provides a confidential support network for homosexual men with various forms of disability, including those associated with ageing. Literature is available on receipt of a sae.

GEMMA
BM Box 5700
London WC1N 3XX

> This organization is concerned with lesbian women of all ages, with and without disabilities.

Hysterectomy Support Group
11 Henryson Road
Brockley
London SE4 1HL Tel. 081-690-5987

> They publish relevant literature, and have self-help groups in various parts of the country.

Ileostomy Association of Great Britain and Ireland
Ambleside House
Black Scotch Lane
Mansfield
Notts NG18 4PF Tel. Mansfield 28099

> The aims and function of this association are similar to the Colostomy Welfare Group.

National Association of Widows
54–57 Allison Street
Digbeth
Birmingham B5 5TH Tel. 021-643-8348

> There are local branches in various parts of the country that provide social support for widows, and information and advice is available by post or telephone.

National Council for the Divorced and Separated
13 High Street
Little Shelford
Cambs. CB2 5ES

> This provides a service similar to that of the National Association of Widows.

National Osteoporosis Society
PO Box 10
Barton Meade House
Radstock
Bath BA3 3YB Tel. 0761-32472

> This society publishes relevant literature, provides information, and has local groups.

Outsiders' Club
Box 4ZB
London W1A Tel. 071-499-0900

This is a support group for physically handicapped people who are seeking to form a relationship.

Parkinson's Disease Society
36 Portland Place
London W1N 3DG Tel. 071-255-2432.
This is similar in its aims and function to the Alzheimer's Disease Society.

Pre-Retirement Association of Great Britain and Northern Ireland
19 Undine Street

Tooting
London SW17 8PP Tel. 081-767-3225.
This provides information about preparation for retirement, including educational courses.

Relate (National Marriage Guidance)
Herbert Gray College
Little Church Street
Rugby CV21 3AP Tel. 0788-73241
Couples of any age can receive marital counselling from the local branch of the Relate Marriage Guidance Council, and health-care professionals should be in touch with these branches.

Standing Conference of Ethnic Minority Senior Citizens
5 Westminster Bridge Road
London SE1 7SW. Tel. 071-928-0095
The special problems of older people in ethnic minorities are considered by this organization, which also promotes community care projects.

University of the Third Age
1 Stockwell Green
London SW9 9JF Tel. 071-737-2541
Throughout the country there are local branches of this organization which runs social, educational and cultural activities for retired people, and those approaching retirement. The above is the address of the co-ordinating office in London, but some of the larger branches are not affiliated; their addresses may be obtained through the local Citizens' Advisory Bureau.

# Author index

# Subject index